GUA SHA FOR ANTI-AGING

Stimulate Collagen, Reduce Wrinkles, and Enhance Your Skin's Youthfulness

George Carolyn

1

Table of Contents

INTRODUCTION

Gua Sha is a traditional healing technique from East Asia, primarily used in Chinese medicine. It involves scraping the skin with a smooth-edged tool, typically made of jade, rose quartz, or other materials, to promote circulation, relieve muscle tension, and improve the flow of energy (qi) throughout the body. While it is commonly used in the context of massage or body therapy, it has recently gained popularity for facial treatments, offering potential benefits like enhanced skin tone, reduced puffiness, and improved elasticity. Applying Gua Sha is a straightforward process, but it requires a gentle touch and understanding of proper technique. When done correctly, it can leave you feeling relaxed and rejuvenated.

Step-by-Step Guide on How to Apply Gua Sha

Choose the Right Tool: Select a Gua Sha tool that suits your needs. For body work, larger tools with a curved edge are ideal. For facial Gua Sha, smaller tools with smooth contours work best.

Jade and rose quartz are popular because they are naturally cooling and believed to have healing properties, but you can also find tools made from stainless steel or other materials.

Prepare Your Skin: Before applying Gua Sha to your skin, make sure your skin is clean and well-moisturized. For facial Gua Sha, apply a few drops of facial oil, serum, or moisturizer. For body work, you can use body lotion, oil, or even coconut oil. The lubrication helps the tool glide smoothly over the skin and prevents irritation.

Start with Gentle Pressure: Begin by holding the Gua Sha tool at a 15–30 degree angle to your skin. You don't need to press too hard; gentle, consistent pressure is sufficient. For facial treatments, a lighter touch is recommended, as the skin on the face is more delicate. For body work, you can apply slightly more pressure to address deeper muscle tension.

Use Long, Sweeping Strokes: The technique involves sweeping the tool along the skin in long, smooth strokes. For the face, start at the center of your face and move outward along the jawline, cheeks, and forehead. Use upward and outward motions to lift the skin. For the body, you can work along the neck, shoulders, back, and limbs, using long strokes in the direction of your lymphatic drainage (toward the heart).

Focus on Tension Areas: When using Gua Sha for muscle tension relief, focus on areas where you feel tightness or discomfort. For example, on the back, shoulders, and neck, use slower, more focused strokes to release knots. On the face, work around areas prone to puffiness, such as under the eyes or along the jawline.

Move Slowly and Methodically: Don't rush through the process. Take your time to apply gentle pressure and ensure you are using smooth, consistent strokes. Each stroke should last 5–10 seconds, and you can repeat each area several times.

Finish with Light Pressure:
After completing the scraping strokes, finish by lightly pressing the tool against your skin for a few seconds to promote relaxation and enhance circulation. This helps the body absorb the benefits of the treatment and can leave your skin feeling more refreshed.

Post-Gua Sha Care:
After your session, it's important to hydrate and take care of your skin. Gua Sha can increase circulation, so be sure to drink plenty of water afterward. For the face, applying a soothing moisturizer or serum will help lock in moisture and support the skin's natural healing process.

Tips for Best Results:

Consistency is key. Regular use of Gua Sha (2–3 times a week) will yield the best results.

Always work in the direction of your lymphatic flow, especially on the face, to promote drainage and avoid irritation.

If you're using Gua Sha for muscle tension, you can apply heat or cold therapy afterward to enhance the treatment.

Avoid using too much pressure. Over-scraping can cause bruising or irritation.

What is Gua Sha?

Gua Sha is a traditional healing technique that originates from Chinese medicine. The name "Gua Sha" translates to "scraping" (Gua) and "sand" (Sha), which refers to the process of scraping the skin with a smooth-edged tool to promote healing and improve circulation. This method has been used for centuries in East Asia to treat various ailments and promote general wellness. While it was initially developed for use on the body to relieve pain, tension, and improve blood flow, Gua Sha has more recently become popular as a beauty treatment, particularly for the face. In this context, it is used to reduce puffiness, enhance skin tone, and improve the overall appearance of the skin.

How Gua Sha Works

The main principle behind Gua Sha is to stimulate blood flow and release muscle tension. When the skin is scraped with the tool, it encourages blood circulation to the area, which helps in removing stagnation, improving the flow of *qi* (vital energy), and aiding in the removal of toxins. This process can reduce inflammation, promote healing, and support the body's natural detoxification processes. In facial treatments, Gua Sha works by stimulating lymphatic drainage, helping to reduce puffiness, enhance skin elasticity, and encourage a glowing complexion.

Common Benefits of Gua Sha

Relieves Muscle Tension: By scraping the skin over sore or tight muscles, Gua Sha helps to release built-up tension and alleviate pain.

Improves Circulation: It encourages better blood flow, which can speed up healing and promote healthier skin.

Reduces Puffiness: Especially in facial treatments, Gua Sha can help to reduce water retention and improve lymphatic drainage, leading to a less puffy appearance.

Promotes Relaxation: The gentle scraping action can induce a calming effect, helping to reduce stress and encourage relaxation.

Improves Skin Tone: Regular use on the face can enhance the appearance of skin by stimulating collagen production and encouraging a firmer, smoother texture.

Tools Used in Gua Sha

Traditionally, Gua Sha was done with tools made from materials like buffalo horn or jade. Nowadays, you'll often find tools made of rose quartz, jade, or stainless steel. These tools come in various shapes and sizes, and the most common ones for facial treatments are shaped like a small, curved "S" or a heart.

The History and Origins of Gua Sha in Traditional Chinese Medicine

Gua Sha is a time-honored technique deeply embedded in the practice of Traditional Chinese Medicine (TCM), with a history that spans thousands of years. Its origins are closely tied to the development of TCM's understanding of the body, energy flow, and healing practices.

Ancient Roots of Gua Sha

The practice of Gua Sha dates back to at least the Tang Dynasty (618-907 AD) in China, though some historians believe it may have been used even earlier, possibly as far back as the Han Dynasty (206 BC–220 AD). In TCM, health and disease are thought to be influenced by the balance and flow of Qi (vital energy) and blood through the body. When Qi stagnates, or blood flow is poor, illness and pain can occur. Gua Sha was developed as a technique to address these imbalances by physically stimulating the skin and muscles to encourage better circulation, the flow of Qi, and the removal of toxins.

Early Gua Sha Tools and Practices

The name "Gua Sha" is derived from two Chinese characters:

"Gua" (刮), which means "scraping" or "rubbing."

"Sha" (痧), which refers to the red marks that can appear on the skin after the scraping, often resembling bruises, and is linked to the term "sand" or "stagnation" in TCM.

Historically, Gua Sha was performed using various tools made from naturally occurring materials such as stone, jade, bone, or horn. The technique was primarily used to treat painful conditions and muscle stiffness, as well as to alleviate fever and cold symptoms. Over time, specialized Gua Sha tools were crafted to ensure smoother and more effective scraping, with stones like jade becoming especially popular due to their believed therapeutic properties.

Gua Sha in Traditional Chinese Medicine

In Traditional Chinese Medicine, Gua Sha is considered a form of external therapy aimed at stimulating the body's meridian system the network of energy pathways that connect different organs. The technique is thought to break up stagnant Qi and blood, facilitating its movement through the body, and is often used for conditions like:

Muscle pain (especially in the back, neck, and shoulders)

Chronic tension

Fever and colds

Headaches

Respiratory issues, like asthma and coughs

A typical Gua Sha session might involve scraping the skin in a specific area (e.g., along the back or shoulders) using a tool with smooth, curved edges. In some cases, practitioners might apply a liniment or herbal ointment to the skin before scraping, as these substances were believed to help with pain relief and Qi circulation.

Gua Sha's Role in TCM Healing Philosophy

The philosophy behind Gua Sha is grounded in the principles of balance and flow. TCM holds that the body's functions are regulated by the harmonious movement of Qi and blood. When Qi or blood stagnates due to external factors (e.g., wind, cold, or dampness) or internal factors (e.g., emotional stress or poor diet), it can lead to pain, disease, or dysfunction. Gua Sha helps address these blockages by promoting the movement of Qi and blood to the affected area, which is believed to relieve pain, reduce inflammation, and encourage healing.

Transition to Modern Uses

While Gua Sha was traditionally practiced in clinical settings by trained TCM practitioners, its uses have evolved. Over time, the technique gained popularity as a self-care practice and became widely known as a beauty and wellness tool. Facial Gua Sha, in particular, has become a mainstream treatment in modern skincare, especially in the West. Facial Gua Sha uses the same principles of stimulating circulation and energy flow but is generally performed with gentler pressure and smaller tools. Instead of treating muscle pain, facial Gua Sha focuses on enhancing skin tone, reducing puffiness, and promoting lymphatic drainage, which has contributed to its rise in popularity within wellness and beauty communities.

Modern-Day Use and Global Popularity

Today, Gua Sha has become a widely recognized treatment both in Eastern and Western wellness practices. In recent years, the technique has gained international recognition, especially in beauty and anti-aging treatments. Many people now use Gua Sha tools for facial massage to reduce wrinkles, dark circles, and puffiness, and to promote glowing skin. At the same time, Gua Sha remains a valuable tool in Traditional Chinese Medicine for pain management and overall health, still practiced in TCM clinics and health centers worldwide. As research continues to explore the benefits of techniques like Gua Sha, it has been increasingly acknowledged for its positive effects on circulation, lymphatic drainage, and pain relief.

The Benefits of Gua Sha for Skin and Health

Gua Sha, a traditional technique with deep roots in Chinese medicine, is not just beneficial for pain relief and muscle tension; it also offers a wide range of benefits for both the skin and overall health. As a holistic therapy, Gua Sha works by stimulating circulation, promoting energy flow, and aiding in the removal of toxins from the body. Below are some of the key health and skincare benefits of Gua Sha:

Benefits of Gua Sha for the Skin

Improves Circulation and Blood Flow

One of the most immediate effects of Gua Sha is increased blood circulation. By gently scraping the skin with a smooth-edged tool, Gua Sha encourages blood flow to the surface of the skin. This enhanced circulation promotes the delivery of nutrients and oxygen to skin cells, contributing to a healthy, radiant complexion.

As a result, regular use of Gua Sha can improve overall skin tone and help brighten the skin, giving it a more youthful and glowing appearance.

Reduces Puffiness and Water Retention

Gua Sha is particularly effective for lymphatic drainage, helping to reduce puffiness in areas prone to water retention, such as the under-eye area and along the jawline. By applying gentle pressure and using upward and outward strokes, Gua Sha stimulates the lymphatic system, encouraging the removal of excess fluid and toxins that can cause swelling and puffiness. This is especially beneficial for those who experience bloating or facial puffiness due to poor circulation or hormonal changes.

Promotes Collagen Production and Skin Firmness

Regular use of Gua Sha on the face can stimulate the production of collagen—a protein essential for skin elasticity and firmness. This is particularly beneficial for those looking to maintain or improve skin's firmness and smoothness. As Gua Sha helps to promote circulation, it also encourages the regeneration of skin cells, making the skin appear firmer and less saggy over time.

Reduces Fine Lines and Wrinkles

By increasing blood flow and stimulating the facial muscles, Gua Sha may help soften the appearance of fine lines and wrinkles. The gentle scraping action encourages skin renewal, which can gradually diminish the visibility of aging signs, such as crow's feet, smile lines, and forehead wrinkles. In addition, the tool's massaging action helps to tone the muscles under the skin, leading to a more lifted and youthful appearance.

Relieves Tension and Promotes Relaxation

The soothing motions of Gua Sha also have a calming effect, helping to reduce muscle tension in the face and neck. This can be especially beneficial for people who experience jaw clenching, TMJ (temporomandibular joint) pain, or facial tension due to stress or anxiety. The release of facial tension can help alleviate headaches and migraines, leading to a sense of relaxation and rejuvenation.

Enhances Product Absorption

Gua Sha helps to promote better absorption of skincare products like serums, oils, and moisturizers. The increased circulation allows these products to penetrate deeper into the skin, maximizing their effectiveness. This makes Gua Sha a great complement to your regular skincare routine.

Health Benefits of Gua Sha

Pain Relief and Muscle Tension Reduction

Historically, Gua Sha was used to relieve muscle pain and tension, particularly in the back, neck, shoulders, and limbs. The scraping motion helps to break up muscle knots and stimulate blood flow to areas of pain or discomfort, offering a natural remedy for sore muscles, stiffness, and tightness. It is often used to treat chronic pain conditions like fibromyalgia, arthritis, and muscle sprains, as it helps alleviate both the pain and inflammation associated with these conditions.

Relieves Headaches and Migraines

Gua Sha is known to be effective for headache relief. By targeting areas of tension in the neck, shoulders, and upper back, it helps alleviate the muscle tightness that often leads to tension headaches and migraines. The increased blood circulation and release of muscle knots can also help prevent future headaches from occurring.

For migraine sufferers, using Gua Sha along the neck and upper back can provide immediate relief from symptoms.

Boosts the Immune System

Gua Sha is also used to boost the immune system by improving circulation and promoting the movement of Qi and blood. In TCM, the practice helps to expel wind, cold, and dampness, which are considered factors that contribute to illness and disease. Gua Sha can be used to treat common cold symptoms, flu, and respiratory issues by stimulating the flow of energy and blood, aiding the body in its natural detoxification processes.

Promotes Lymphatic Drainage and Detoxification

Gua Sha's scraping motion encourages the movement of lymph fluid, which helps to remove toxins from the body and improve the immune system's ability to fight off illness.

Lymphatic drainage can also contribute to a reduction in swelling and inflammation, which is beneficial for overall health and well-being.

Improves Flexibility and Range of Motion

By breaking up muscle adhesions and promoting the flow of blood, Gua Sha can improve joint mobility and flexibility. It's often used as part of rehabilitation or recovery for sports injuries and muscle strain, as it helps to speed up healing and reduce recovery time. Regular practice can be beneficial for those with conditions like sciatica, frozen shoulder, and lower back pain, as it helps to release tight muscles and restore movement.

Enhances Relaxation and Reduces Stress

Gua Sha has a relaxing effect on the nervous system, reducing stress and promoting a feeling of calm. The gentle scraping stimulates the parasympathetic nervous system, which is responsible for relaxation and healing. This makes Gua Sha an excellent therapy for managing stress, anxiety, and promoting overall mental well-being.

Why You Should Use Gua Sha: Beauty, Wellness, and Relaxation

Gua Sha, an ancient practice rooted in Traditional Chinese Medicine (TCM), has become a popular wellness and beauty treatment, offering a natural and holistic approach to maintaining health, beauty, and relaxation. Whether you're looking to enhance your skin's appearance, alleviate muscle tension, or de-stress after a busy day, Gua Sha can be a powerful addition to your self-care routine. Here's why you should consider incorporating Gua Sha into your lifestyle:

1. Natural Skin Rejuvenation and Glow

One of the most notable benefits of Gua Sha is its positive impact on the skin. Regular use can leave your skin looking refreshed, brighter, and more youthful. Here's how Gua Sha enhances your skin:

Stimulates Circulation: The scraping motion promotes blood flow, bringing more oxygen and nutrients to the skin. This enhanced circulation helps to revitalize the complexion, making it appear more radiant and healthy.

Boosts Collagen Production: Gua Sha helps stimulate collagen and elastin production, which are essential for skin elasticity and firmness. This can help reduce the appearance of sagging, fine lines, and wrinkles, contributing to a more toned and youthful look.

Reduces Puffiness and Swelling: By encouraging lymphatic drainage, Gua Sha helps to eliminate excess fluid and toxins from the skin, which can reduce puffiness, especially around the eyes and along the jawline. This makes it an excellent tool for combating morning bloating and facial puffiness.

Improves Skin Texture: Gua Sha helps to smooth out rough skin and reduce the appearance of blemishes, acne scars, and hyperpigmentation. The enhanced circulation supports better skin renewal and healing.

Using Gua Sha regularly can enhance the glow and health of your skin in a completely natural way, without the need for harsh chemicals or invasive procedures.

2. Relieves Stress and Promotes Relaxation

In today's fast-paced world, stress is inevitable, but finding ways to manage it is essential for maintaining both mental and physical health. Gua Sha provides a therapeutic approach to relaxation:

Stimulates the Parasympathetic Nervous System: The act of scraping your skin with a Gua Sha tool has a calming effect on the nervous system. It activates the parasympathetic nervous system, which is responsible for promoting relaxation and recovery. This helps reduce overall stress levels, promoting feelings of peace and calm.

Reduces Muscle Tension: Tension often builds up in the muscles, particularly around the neck, shoulders, and jawline, as a response to stress. Gua Sha effectively relieves these tensions, helping to soften tight muscles and reduce discomfort. This can be especially beneficial for those who suffer from chronic tension or TMJ (temporomandibular joint disorder).

Promotes Better Sleep: By calming the nervous system and relaxing the muscles, Gua Sha can contribute to better quality sleep. Many people find that using Gua Sha in the evening, particularly on the face and neck, helps to relieve the stress accumulated during the day, preparing the body for a restful night.

3. Alleviates Muscle Pain and Improves Flexibility

Gua Sha has long been used in TCM to treat pain and promote healing. When it comes to muscle soreness, joint stiffness, or chronic discomfort, Gua Sha offers a natural, drug-free alternative to pain relief:

Relieves Chronic Pain: Gua Sha is effective in easing chronic muscle pain and tension, especially in areas like the back, shoulders, and neck. The technique helps break up muscle adhesions, improve blood flow, and increase flexibility. This makes it ideal for individuals with fibromyalgia, arthritis, or those experiencing chronic muscle tightness due to sedentary lifestyles or stress.

Increases Range of Motion: Regular use of Gua Sha can help improve flexibility and increase the range of motion in stiff joints and muscles. This is particularly helpful for athletes or people recovering from injuries, as it helps to speed up recovery and prevent further muscle stiffness.

Post-Exercise Recovery: Gua Sha is often used after physical activity to soothe sore muscles and speed up the healing process. By improving circulation and reducing muscle inflammation, it aids in quicker recovery and can reduce the chance of injury in the future.

4. Promotes Lymphatic Drainage and Detoxification

One of the key health benefits of Gua Sha is its ability to promote lymphatic drainage, which helps rid the body of toxins and waste products. Here's how this works:

Helps Detoxify the Body: The scraping technique stimulates the lymphatic system, which is responsible for transporting lymph, a fluid that contains white blood cells that fight infection and remove waste from the body. When the lymphatic system is functioning optimally, it aids in detoxifying the body and boosting overall health.

Reduces Inflammation: By improving lymphatic flow, Gua Sha helps to reduce inflammation throughout the body. This is beneficial for individuals suffering from conditions like swelling, edema, or inflammatory skin issues like acne or eczema.

Improves Immune Function: An optimally functioning lymphatic system plays a key role in supporting immune health. Regular Gua Sha can help enhance your immune system's ability to ward off illness and reduce the frequency of colds and infections.

5. Simple, Non-Invasive, and Affordable

One of the biggest advantages of Gua Sha is that it's a non-invasive, affordable, and simple technique that can be done in the comfort of your own home. Unlike expensive spa treatments or invasive cosmetic procedures, Gua Sha is a safe and accessible option for improving your skin health and general well-being.

Easy to Learn and Use: Gua Sha is relatively simple to master, especially for facial treatments. There are numerous tutorials and guides available, and with just a few tools (typically a jade, rose quartz, or stainless-steel scraper), you can begin incorporating it into your daily routine.

Minimal Side Effects: Gua Sha has very few risks when used properly. While temporary red marks (called sha) can appear on the skin, they typically fade within a few hours to a day, indicating that blood flow has been improved in the area.

Affordable Self-Care: Gua Sha tools can be purchased for a relatively low cost, making it an affordable alternative to high-priced beauty treatments and therapies.

6. Supports Overall Wellness

Beyond beauty and relaxation, Gua Sha supports overall physical health by addressing issues like chronic pain, poor circulation, and low energy. Here's why it contributes to your general wellness:

Balances Energy (Qi): According to TCM, the flow of Qi is essential for overall health. When Qi becomes blocked or stagnates, it can lead to pain, fatigue, and illness. Gua Sha helps release blockages, encouraging the free flow of energy throughout the body.

Helps with Digestion and Bloating: Gua Sha is also used to treat digestive issues by stimulating the abdomen and promoting better circulation in the digestive organs. It can help reduce bloating and alleviate constipation, improving overall digestive health.

Supports Mental Health: As a form of self-care, Gua Sha can enhance feelings of well-being and calm. By reducing stress, alleviating tension, and promoting relaxation, it supports a healthier, more balanced mental state.

What to Expect from This Book: A Guide to Gua Sha for Beauty, Wellness, and Relaxation

Welcome to a transformative journey into the world of Gua Sha an ancient healing practice with profound benefits for both your skin and overall well-being. This book is designed to provide you with all the knowledge, tools, and techniques you need to incorporate Gua Sha into your daily routine, unlocking its powerful potential for beauty, wellness, and relaxation.

Here's what you can expect from this book:

1. A Comprehensive Introduction to Gua Sha

Origins and History: Learn about the rich history and cultural significance of Gua Sha in Traditional Chinese Medicine (TCM), dating back thousands of years. Discover how this ancient practice has evolved and found its place in modern wellness and skincare routines.

The Science Behind Gua Sha: Understand the physiological effects of Gua Sha on the body, including how it promotes blood circulation, stimulates lymphatic drainage, and aids in the natural detoxification process.

2. In-Depth Exploration of Gua Sha Benefits

For Beauty: Learn how Gua Sha can help improve your complexion by stimulating collagen production, reducing puffiness, and promoting a radiant, glowing appearance. This book delves into the benefits of facial Gua Sha for reducing wrinkles, enhancing skin elasticity, and improving skin texture.

For Wellness: Explore how Gua Sha alleviates muscle tension, promotes flexibility, and provides relief from chronic pain. You'll learn about its role in improving circulation, reducing inflammation, and helping with conditions like headaches, muscle stiffness, and joint pain.

For Relaxation: Discover how the rhythmic, soothing motions of Gua Sha can relax your mind and body, reduce stress, and help you unwind. Understand its connection to mental well-being and how it can promote better sleep and emotional balance.

3. Step-by-Step Guides and Techniques

How to Use Gua Sha Tools: Detailed instructions on how to use various Gua Sha tools, including jade, rose quartz, and stainless steel, for both facial and body treatments. Learn the proper techniques for effective scraping, pressure, and strokes.

Facial Gua Sha Routine: Step-by-step guides to facial Gua Sha, targeting specific areas like the forehead, jawline, cheeks, and under the eyes. You'll also find tips for using Gua Sha in combination with your favorite serums or oils for maximum benefit.

Body Gua Sha for Muscle Pain: Learn how to use Gua Sha on the back, shoulders, neck, and other parts of the body to relieve muscle tension, alleviate soreness, and promote healing.

4. Tips and Troubleshooting

How to Achieve the Best Results: Gain insights on how often to practice Gua Sha, what products to use, and how to incorporate it into your wellness routine for maximum effectiveness.

Troubleshooting Common Mistakes: Avoid common pitfalls, such as using too much pressure, improper angles, or incorrect techniques, by following easy-to-understand tips and solutions.

Safety Precautions: Learn the safety guidelines for using Gua Sha, especially when applying it to sensitive areas or dealing with specific skin conditions.

5. Advanced Gua Sha Practices

Gua Sha for Specific Conditions: Delve deeper into how Gua Sha can be tailored for specific health conditions, such as relieving chronic pain, improving lymphatic drainage, and treating issues like sinus congestion or digestive problems.

Combining Gua Sha with Other Therapies: Understand how Gua Sha can complement other wellness practices, like acupressure, aromatherapy, or yoga, to enhance its healing effects.

6. Mindfulness and the Holistic Approach

Gua Sha as a Self-Care Ritual: Learn how to turn your Gua Sha practice into a mindful, restorative ritual that goes beyond beauty and health. Embrace the calming effects of slow, deliberate movements to connect with yourself and cultivate a deeper sense of relaxation and presence.

The Importance of Self-Love: Explore how incorporating Gua Sha into your routine can boost your mental and emotional well-being, helping you foster a greater sense of self-care, self-love, and body positivity.

7. Personal Stories and Testimonials

Real-Life Experiences: Hear from people who have incorporated Gua Sha into their lives and experienced transformative results. From improved skin appearance to relief from chronic pain, their stories offer inspiration and insights on how Gua Sha can become a life-changing practice.

Guided Success Stories: Learn from testimonials about how Gua Sha has enhanced people's beauty routines, helped them recover from injuries, and brought them greater physical and emotional well-being.

8. Resources for Further Learning

Where to Buy Gua Sha Tools: Find out where to purchase high-quality Gua Sha tools, and what to look for when choosing the right one for your needs.

Further Reading and References: Explore books, articles, and studies for those who want to dive deeper into the theory and science behind Gua Sha and its connection to traditional Chinese healing practices.

CHAPTER ONE

GETTING STARTED WITH GUA SHA

Welcome to the world of Gua Sha! In this chapter, we will guide you through the essential steps to ensure you're ready to experience the full benefits of this powerful technique. From understanding the different types of Gua Sha tools to preparing your skin and setting the right environment, this chapter will lay the foundation for your Gua Sha practice. We'll also highlight important safety tips to ensure you avoid common mistakes, so you can use Gua Sha safely and effectively.

UNDERSTANDING GUA SHA TOOLS: TYPES AND MATERIALS

The right Gua Sha tool can make all the difference in your practice. Tools come in various shapes, sizes, and materials, each serving different purposes. Here's a breakdown of the most popular types of Gua Sha tools and the materials they are made from:

1. Stone Gua Sha Tools

Traditionally, Gua Sha tools were made from stones, which were believed to carry certain healing properties. The most common stones used include:

Jade: A highly revered stone in Traditional Chinese Medicine, jade is known for its cool, soothing properties and ability to promote healing. It is believed to balance the body's energy and calm inflammation.

Rose Quartz: Known as the stone of love, rose quartz is said to have gentle, healing properties that help reduce stress and promote relaxation. It's a great choice for those who want to enhance their skincare routine with a calming, emotional boost.

Amethyst: This crystal is known for its purifying energy and is often chosen for its calming effect, helping to reduce stress and promote relaxation during Gua Sha sessions.

2. Stainless Steel Gua Sha Tools

Stainless steel Gua Sha tools have become increasingly popular in recent years. They are durable, easy to clean, and provide a smooth, consistent scraping experience. Unlike stone tools, stainless steel is often favored for its practicality and ability to retain a uniform temperature, which is essential for specific therapeutic uses.

Benefits: Stainless steel tools are less likely to absorb oils or lotions, which makes them ideal for hygiene-conscious users. They're also easy to sterilize and more lightweight compared to stone options.

3. Other Materials

In addition to jade, rose quartz, and stainless steel, some Gua Sha tools are made from materials like horn (often water buffalo or ox horn) and bamboo. These materials are less common but are still used in certain traditional practices.

CHOOSING THE RIGHT GUA SHA TOOL FOR YOUR NEEDS

The best Gua Sha tool for you will depend on your personal preferences, skin type, and the specific benefits you're seeking. Here's how to choose the right tool based on your needs:

For Facial Use:

Jade and Rose Quartz Tools: If you're focused on facial Gua Sha, look for tools that are specifically designed for delicate areas like the under-eyes, forehead, and jawline. These tools typically have a more curved shape, allowing for precise movements and gentle pressure.

Small, Contoured Tools: For the face, you'll want tools that are small and have a contoured design to fit the natural curves of your face, especially around the eyes and nose.

For Body Use:

Larger, Flat Tools: For larger areas like your back, shoulders, or legs, opt for a bigger, flatter tool that can cover more surface area. These tools often have more pronounced edges to apply deeper pressure.

Stainless Steel: If you're seeking a tool for both facial and body use and want something versatile and easy to clean, a stainless steel tool might be ideal.

For Sensitivity or First-Time Users:

Gentler Stones: If you're new to Gua Sha or have sensitive skin, opt for a rose quartz or jade tool, as these stones are generally considered softer and more soothing.

Flat, Rounded Tools: Choose a tool with soft, rounded edges to avoid any harsh scraping that might irritate the skin, especially if you have sensitive or reactive skin.

PREPARING YOUR SKIN FOR GUA SHA: CLEANSING AND HYDRATION

Before you begin your Gua Sha practice, it's important to prepare your skin to ensure that it's clean, hydrated, and ready for the treatment. Here's how to properly prepare:

1. Cleanse Your Skin Thoroughly

Start with a gentle facial cleanser that suits your skin type. The goal is to remove any dirt, oil, or makeup so that the Gua Sha tool can glide smoothly over your skin without causing any irritation. If you're using Gua Sha on your body, take a warm shower beforehand to cleanse your skin and soften any muscle tension.

2. Hydrate and Add a Slip

Gua Sha requires some form of lubrication to ensure the tool glides smoothly over your skin without dragging or pulling. Here's what to use:

Facial Oil or Serum: Choose a nourishing facial oil or serum that is appropriate for your skin type. Rosehip oil, jojoba oil, and argan oil are great options for hydration and nourishment.

Body Oil or Lotion: If you're using Gua Sha on your body, apply a generous amount of body oil or lotion to the area you'll be working on. This will provide enough slip for the tool to move effortlessly across the skin.

CREATING THE RIGHT ENVIRONMENT: SETTING UP YOUR SPACE

Creating a peaceful and relaxing environment is key to enjoying your Gua Sha session. Here are some tips to enhance your experience:

1. Choose a Calm Space

Find a quiet, comfortable space where you can relax without distractions. Whether it's your bedroom, bathroom, or a cozy corner of your home, ensure it's a space where you feel at ease.

2. Set the Mood with Lighting and Aromatherapy

Lighting: Use soft, ambient lighting to set the tone. Dim the lights or use candles to create a calming atmosphere.

Aromatherapy: Diffuse calming essential oils like lavender, chamomile, or eucalyptus. The right scent can help you relax and enhance the therapeutic benefits of Gua Sha.

3. Comfortable Positioning

When performing facial Gua Sha, sit or recline in a comfortable position, ideally with a mirror in front of you. For body Gua Sha, you might prefer lying down or sitting comfortably in a chair, depending on the area you are working on.

GUA SHA SAFETY TIPS: HOW TO AVOID COMMON MISTAKES

While Gua Sha is generally safe, it's important to follow some basic guidelines to avoid injury and ensure that you're using the technique properly. Here are some essential safety tips:

1. Don't Apply Too Much Pressure

One of the most common mistakes beginners make is using excessive pressure during their Gua Sha session. While Gua Sha should feel therapeutic, it should not be painful.

Use light to moderate pressure, especially on the face. The tool should glide smoothly over the skin, not drag or tug. Adjust the pressure based on your comfort level.

2. Avoid Scraping Over Bony Areas

Be gentle around bony parts of the body, such as the cheekbones, forehead, and jawline. Applying too much pressure on these areas can cause discomfort or bruising.

3. Keep the Tool Clean

Always clean your Gua Sha tool before and after use to avoid introducing bacteria to your skin. Simply wash it with warm water and mild soap, and dry it thoroughly. If you use oils or serums, wipe the tool down after each session to remove any residue.

4. Don't Overdo It

Gua Sha is a powerful technique, but it's important not to overdo it. Limit your facial Gua Sha sessions to around 5-10 minutes, and body sessions to 10-15 minutes, depending on your comfort and the area you're targeting.

Avoid daily Gua Sha on sensitive areas, as excessive scraping can lead to irritation. Start by using the technique 2-3 times a week and increase frequency as your skin gets accustomed.

5. Know When to Avoid Gua Sha

If you have skin conditions like open wounds, sunburn, or active acne, avoid using Gua Sha on affected areas. Gua Sha can be too intense for sensitive skin or inflamed conditions. If you have blood clotting disorders or are on blood thinners, consult with a healthcare provider before using Gua Sha, as the scraping can promote circulation and may not be suitable for certain medical conditions.

CHAPTER TWO

THE BASIC TECHNIQUE – STEP-BY-STEP GUIDE

In this chapter, we will guide you through the essential techniques for using your Gua Sha tool effectively. Mastering the correct grip, pressure, angles, and motions is key to ensuring that your Gua Sha practice is both safe and beneficial. Once you have a solid understanding of these basic techniques, you'll be able to incorporate Gua Sha into your routine with confidence, achieving the desired beauty and wellness benefits.

HOW TO HOLD YOUR GUA SHA TOOL CORRECTLY

The way you hold your Gua Sha tool is crucial to ensuring both comfort and effectiveness during your practice. Here's how to grip the tool properly:

1. Grip with Your Fingers, Not Your Palm

Hold the tool with a relaxed grip, using your fingers rather than your palm. The tool should rest comfortably between your fingers, allowing your hand to maintain a flexible and fluid movement.

Avoid squeezing the tool tightly; a loose but controlled grip is ideal.

2. Tool Positioning

For facial Gua Sha, keep the tool at a slight angle (about 15-30 degrees) to your skin. This allows the edge of the tool to make proper contact without dragging or causing discomfort.

For body Gua Sha, the tool should be held slightly flatter, depending on the size of the area you are working on. Keep the edge of the tool against the skin, applying even pressure as you glide.

PROPER PRESSURE AND ANGLES FOR EFFECTIVE GUA SHA

The effectiveness of your Gua Sha practice relies heavily on applying the correct pressure and using the right angles. Here's how to find that sweet spot:

1. Apply Light to Moderate Pressure

Gua Sha should never feel painful. The pressure should be enough to feel the scraping sensation, but not so intense that it causes discomfort or leaves lasting marks. On the face, especially, you should use gentle pressure, with the goal of stimulating circulation without irritating the skin.

For Facial Gua Sha: Light pressure is best. The skin on your face is more delicate, and heavy pressure can lead to redness or bruising.

For Body Gua Sha: You can apply moderate pressure, especially in areas of muscle tension. The skin on your back, neck, and shoulders is thicker, so a bit more pressure can be applied here.

2. The Correct Angles

Facial Application: Hold the tool at a 15-30 degree angle to the skin. This allows the tool to glide smoothly across the surface without dragging. The edge should make gentle contact with your skin, with the flat side of the tool resting lightly on the surface.

Body Application: For larger body areas (such as the back or thighs), a more horizontal angle is appropriate. The edge of the tool should lie flat against the skin to cover a broader area.

Mastering the Basic Strokes for Facial and Neck Application

Once you're comfortable with the tool and pressure, it's time to start incorporating strokes. There are several basic strokes used in facial Gua Sha that help promote circulation, stimulate lymphatic drainage, and provide muscle relief.

1. Forehead Strokes

How to do it: Start at the center of your forehead, right between your eyebrows, and gently glide the tool upward towards your hairline. Use long, smooth strokes.

Angle: Hold the tool at a 15-30 degree angle to the skin.

Pressure: Light to moderate pressure.

Purpose: This helps reduce tension in the forehead and improves circulation, promoting a smoother, less furrowed brow.

2. Eye Area

How to do it: Start from the inner corner of your eyebrow and glide the tool out towards the temple. Be very gentle around the delicate under-eye area, using light strokes.

Angle: Keep the tool slightly more vertical here to target the soft skin under the eyes.

Pressure: Very light pressure. This area is sensitive, so it's important to be gentle.

Purpose: Gua Sha on this area helps reduce puffiness, smooth fine lines, and promote lymphatic drainage.

3. Cheeks and Jawline

How to do it: Starting from the nose, glide the tool across the cheekbones toward the ear. Follow this with gentle strokes along the jawline, from chin to ear, helping to define the jaw and stimulate circulation.

Angle: Maintain a 15-30 degree angle to your skin.

Pressure: Light to moderate pressure for the cheeks, but you can use slightly more pressure on the jawline.

Purpose: These strokes enhance circulation, reduce puffiness, and promote facial contouring.

4. Neck Strokes

How to do it: From the base of the neck, gently glide the tool upward towards the jawline. You can also use upward strokes along the sides of your neck, following the natural lines of your muscles.

Angle: The tool should be at a shallow angle (around 15-20 degrees) when gliding upward.

Pressure: Light pressure. The neck is a sensitive area, so avoid heavy pressure.

Purpose: These strokes promote lymphatic drainage, reduce tension in the neck, and help define the jawline.

THE ESSENTIAL MOTIONS: GLIDING, SCRAPING, AND LIFTING

Gua Sha involves three main motions: gliding, scraping, and lifting. Each motion serves a distinct purpose and should be used with intention.

1. Gliding

What it is: Gliding is the continuous, smooth movement of the Gua Sha tool along the skin. This motion is often used for lymphatic drainage, as it helps move fluids toward the lymph nodes.

How to do it: Hold the tool at a slight angle, and glide it in long, continuous strokes. Keep the pressure light and the tool moving smoothly across the skin.

When to use it: Gliding is used in almost every stroke for facial and body applications, particularly for improving circulation and lymphatic drainage.

2. Scraping

What it is: Scraping involves using more direct, focused pressure to break up tension, adhesions, or stagnation in the muscles or tissues. Scraping is typically deeper than gliding but should still feel comfortable.

How to do it: Scrape the tool firmly over areas of tightness, such as the shoulders, neck, or back. The movement should be slower and deliberate. Make sure to maintain the tool's contact with the skin without causing pain.

When to use it: Scraping is effective on muscle areas that are tense, sore, or need deeper stimulation. For example, the neck or back may benefit from scraping.

3. Lifting

What it is: Lifting involves using the edge of the Gua Sha tool to lift and stimulate the muscles, particularly in the face. This motion is particularly beneficial for facial toning and muscle relaxation.

How to do it: After gliding the tool along a section of the face or body, gently lift the tool at the end of each stroke, as if you're pulling the skin upward.

When to use it: Use lifting motions along the jawline and cheekbones to help promote a lifted, sculpted look. It's particularly effective for areas with sagging or muscle tightness.

UNDERSTANDING THE DIRECTION OF STROKES AND THEIR IMPACT ON THE SKIN

The direction of your strokes is crucial for achieving the intended benefits of Gua Sha. Here's how to understand the impact of different directions:

1. Upward Strokes

Why they're important: Upward strokes help lift and tone the skin, particularly in areas like the jawline, cheeks, and forehead. They are essential for counteracting the natural downward pull of gravity and promoting a more sculpted appearance.

Where to use them: On the cheeks, jawline, neck, and forehead, aiming to lift the skin and promote circulation.

2. Outward Strokes

Why they're important: Outward strokes are effective for stimulating lymphatic drainage. Moving fluid away from the center of the face toward the temples helps clear toxins and reduces puffiness, especially around the eyes and jaw.

Where to use them: From the center of the forehead, nose, or chin outward toward the temples or ears.

3. Downward Strokes

Why they're important: While most strokes should be upward or outward, downward strokes can be useful for areas like the neck. Moving downward can help promote lymphatic drainage towards the lymph nodes located in the neck area.

Where to use them: On the neck and collarbone area, moving downward to encourage lymphatic drainage.

CHAPTER THREE

GUA SHA FOR FACIAL REJUVENATION

Gua Sha isn't just an ancient therapy for overall well-being it's also a powerful tool for facial rejuvenation, offering natural, non-invasive solutions to a variety of skin concerns. In this chapter, we will dive deep into the ways Gua Sha enhances your skin's appearance, improves circulation, and helps tone and lift the face. Whether you're aiming to reduce puffiness, sculpt your jawline, or reduce fine lines and wrinkles, Gua Sha can be a transformative addition to your skincare routine.

HOW GUA SHA IMPROVES BLOOD CIRCULATION AND LYMPHATIC DRAINAGE

The foundation of facial rejuvenation with Gua Sha lies in its ability to improve both blood circulation and lymphatic drainage, which are essential for healthy, glowing skin. Let's explore how these two mechanisms work together to support your skin's natural radiance.

1. Blood Circulation

Boosts Oxygen and Nutrients: Gua Sha's scraping motion stimulates the skin and underlying tissues, encouraging increased blood flow to the area. Enhanced circulation helps deliver more oxygen and nutrients to the skin cells, resulting in a healthier, more vibrant complexion.

Faster Skin Healing: Improved blood circulation speeds up the removal of waste products like carbon dioxide and lactic acid from your skin cells, promoting quicker skin regeneration and healing.

Glow and Radiance: As blood flow improves, you'll notice a more rosy, youthful glow to your skin. This is especially noticeable on areas like the cheeks and forehead, where blood circulation tends to be slower.

2. Lymphatic Drainage

Reduces Fluid Retention: The lymphatic system is responsible for removing toxins and waste from the body.

By stimulating lymphatic drainage, Gua Sha helps reduce fluid retention, which can lead to puffiness and a sluggish complexion.

Detoxification: Gua Sha encourages the movement of lymph fluids towards the lymph nodes, helping to flush out toxins and waste products from the skin. This can help reduce breakouts, dullness, and promote clearer skin.

Slimming Effect: As the lymphatic system is stimulated, you may also notice a subtle slimming effect on the face, especially around the jawline and cheeks, as excess fluid is eliminated.

TARGET AREAS FOR FACIAL TONING AND LIFTING

Gua Sha is particularly effective at toning and lifting specific areas of the face, where muscles and skin can become lax over time due to aging, stress, or poor circulation. Understanding the target areas for facial lifting will help you achieve the sculpted, rejuvenated look you desire.

1. Cheeks and Nasolabial Folds

Toning the Cheeks: Regular Gua Sha on the cheeks promotes toning and muscle stimulation, which helps prevent sagging and encourages a fuller, plumper appearance.

Treating Nasolabial Folds: The deep lines that run from the nose to the corners of the mouth (known as nasolabial folds) can be softened with gentle Gua Sha strokes. Focus on the area under the cheekbones and around the corners of the mouth to smooth and lift these lines.

2. Jawline and Neck

Sculpting the Jawline: The jawline area is often one of the first to show signs of sagging as we age. Gua Sha can help lift and define the jawline by stimulating the muscles and tissues.

Neck Toning: Gua Sha is also effective for toning the neck area, where skin can become loose. Gently scrape upward along the neck to encourage a firmer, more defined neckline.

3. Forehead

Lift the Forehead: Gua Sha works wonders on the forehead, particularly to smooth out lines caused by stress or repetitive facial expressions. The gentle upward strokes help lift the brow area, giving the face a more open, refreshed look.

REDUCING PUFFINESS: GUA SHA FOR UNDER-EYE CIRCLES

Puffy eyes and under-eye circles are common concerns for many people, whether caused by lack of sleep, allergies, or fluid retention. Gua Sha can be incredibly effective in reducing puffiness and rejuvenating the delicate skin around the eyes.

1. The Role of Lymphatic Drainage in Puffiness

The skin under the eyes is delicate and prone to fluid buildup. By gently stimulating the lymphatic system, Gua

Sha encourages the movement of stagnant fluid, which helps reduce puffiness. This is especially helpful if you wake up with swollen eyes or if you have chronic under-eye puffiness.

2. The Right Technique

Gentle, Light Pressure: The skin around the eyes is thin and sensitive, so it's important to use light pressure when performing Gua Sha here. You don't want to drag or pull the skin; instead, focus on gentle, gliding motions.

Technique: Start at the inner corner of the eye, near the tear duct, and gently glide the Gua Sha tool out toward the temples, following the natural line of the orbital bone. You can repeat this on both the upper and lower eyelids to promote lymphatic drainage and reduce fluid retention.

3. Combining with Eye Creams or Serums

For added benefit, apply a nourishing eye cream or serum before performing Gua Sha on the under-eye area. The cream will provide additional hydration and nourishment while allowing the tool to glide more easily. Ingredients like caffeine, hyaluronic acid, and peptides can help reduce puffiness and support skin regeneration.

SCULPTING THE JAWLINE AND CHEEKS WITH GUA SHA

One of the most sought-after benefits of Gua Sha is its ability to sculpt and define the jawline and cheekbones, areas that are often prone to puffiness or sagging as we age. Let's explore how Gua Sha can help you achieve a more sculpted face.

1. Defining the Jawline

Lift and Firm: Start by placing the tool at the center of the chin and gently glide it along the jawline toward the ears. This motion helps reduce fluid retention and tension, allowing the jawline to appear more sharp and defined.

Toning the Muscles: The scraping motion also helps tone the underlying muscles in the jaw, providing subtle lifting effects over time. It can also aid in reducing tension or tightness in the muscles around the jaw, making it an excellent remedy for those who grind their teeth or suffer from jaw clenching.

2. Sculpting the Cheeks

Lift and Plump: Focus on lifting the skin from the cheekbones upward toward the temples. This helps counteract gravity and enhance the natural structure of the face. With consistent use, Gua Sha can help give the cheeks a plumper, more youthful appearance.

Chisel the Cheeks: By scraping along the edges of the cheekbones, Gua Sha can subtly enhance the appearance of the bone structure, making your cheeks look more sculpted and defined.

GUA SHA FOR WRINKLE REDUCTION: STIMULATING COLLAGEN PRODUCTION

One of the most remarkable benefits of Gua Sha is its ability to stimulate collagen production, which helps reduce the appearance of wrinkles and fine lines. Regular

Gua Sha practice can promote skin regeneration and lead to smoother, more youthful-looking skin.

1. Collagen Production and Skin Renewal

Collagen Stimulation: The mechanical scraping action of Gua Sha stimulates the skin and underlying tissues, encouraging the production of collagen and elastin, proteins that are essential for maintaining the skin's structure and elasticity. Increased collagen leads to firmer, more supple skin, reducing the appearance of fine lines and wrinkles.

2. Focus Areas for Wrinkle Reduction

Forehead Lines: For horizontal lines on the forehead, use gentle upward strokes with the tool. This helps improve blood flow and encourages collagen production in the area.

Crow's Feet: For fine lines around the eyes, use very light, circular motions along the outer corners. This stimulates the skin and encourages the formation of new, healthy skin cells.

Smile Lines: The nasolabial folds (smile lines) can be softened by gently scraping from the corners of the nose to the mouth and then out toward the temples.

CHAPTER FOUR

GUA SHA FOR SKIN CARE AND MAXIMIZING RESULTS

Gua Sha can be an incredibly powerful addition to your skincare routine, enhancing the effects of your favorite products and offering deeper rejuvenation. To make the most of your Gua Sha practice, it's important to combine it with the right skincare products and techniques. Whether you're trying to boost hydration, target acne, or maintain a clear, glowing complexion, this chapter will guide you on how to maximize your Gua Sha results and tailor your routine for your specific skin needs.

ENHANCING YOUR ROUTINE: PAIRING GUA SHA WITH SERUMS AND OILS

The benefits of Gua Sha are greatly amplified when combined with the right skincare products. Serums and oils provide the perfect slip for the Gua Sha tool, allowing it to glide smoothly across the skin while nourishing and hydrating at a deeper level.

1. The Importance of Pairing Gua Sha with Hydrating Products

Better Absorption: When applied before Gua Sha, hydrating serums and oils help the product penetrate deeper into the skin, enhancing its efficacy. The tool helps push the product into the skin while simultaneously stimulating blood circulation.

Increased Moisture: Many oils and serums contain ingredients that lock moisture into the skin. By using Gua Sha on top of these products, you help create a barrier that seals in hydration, preventing moisture loss throughout the day or night.

2. How to Pair Gua Sha with Skincare Products

Cleansing: Always begin with a clean face to ensure the tool doesn't drag or irritate the skin. Cleanse using a gentle facial cleanser.

Toning: After cleansing, apply a toner or essence to hydrate and balance the skin's pH.

Serum/Oil Application: Apply a generous layer of serum or oil to the face and neck. This is where you can tailor your choice of products based on your skin's specific needs. Next, use the Gua Sha tool to perform your facial massage, allowing the product to absorb more effectively. By pairing Gua Sha with these products, you'll create a synergistic skincare routine that maximizes the benefits of both the tool and the skincare ingredients.

THE BEST FACIAL OILS FOR GUA SHA APPLICATION

Choosing the right facial oil is crucial when incorporating Gua Sha into your skincare routine. The oil you select should have the right consistency to allow the tool to glide smoothly over the skin without dragging or causing irritation.

1. Jojoba Oil

Benefits: Jojoba oil is incredibly versatile and suitable for all skin types. It closely mimics the skin's natural sebum, making it an excellent choice for balancing the skin's oil production. Jojoba oil is light yet nourishing and provides the perfect slip for Gua Sha.

Best for: Dry, combination, or oily skin. It helps regulate sebum and provides hydration without clogging pores.

2. Rosehip Oil

Benefits: Rich in vitamins A, C, and essential fatty acids, rosehip oil is renowned for its anti-aging properties. It promotes skin regeneration and brightening, making it an excellent option for those with fine lines, hyperpigmentation, or dull skin.

Best for: Mature skin, hyperpigmentation, acne scars, and fine lines.

3. Argan Oil

Benefits: Known for its moisturizing and anti-inflammatory properties, argan oil is rich in vitamin E and essential fatty acids. It helps maintain skin elasticity and softness, making it perfect for dry or aging skin.

Best for: Dry, sensitive, or aging skin. Argan oil helps improve skin tone and texture while nourishing and softening the skin.

4. Squalane

Benefits: Squalane is a lightweight, non-comedogenic oil derived from olive oil or sugarcane. It hydrates deeply and improves the skin's barrier function. Its lightweight texture makes it a great option for Gua Sha, as it doesn't feel too greasy but still provides excellent slip.

Best for: Oily, acne-prone, and dehydrated skin. It's especially useful for keeping the skin hydrated without clogging pores.

5. Lavender or Chamomile Infused Oils

Benefits: Infused oils like lavender or chamomile are perfect for calming and soothing irritated or inflamed skin. These oils also provide anti-aging and antioxidant benefits.

Best for: Sensitive or reactive skin. Lavender oil also promotes relaxation, making it a wonderful addition to a nighttime Gua Sha routine.

USING GUA SHA FOR ACNE-PRONE SKIN: BENEFITS AND CAUTIONS

While Gua Sha can be an excellent way to support skin health, those with acne-prone skin must be cautious in how they incorporate it into their routine. The right approach can help reduce inflammation and promote lymphatic drainage, but there are important considerations to keep in mind.

1. How Gua Sha Helps Acne-Prone Skin

Lymphatic Drainage: One of the primary benefits of Gua Sha for acne-prone skin is its ability to encourage lymphatic drainage, helping to reduce puffiness and fluid retention that can exacerbate acne.

Improved Circulation: By boosting blood flow, Gua Sha can help deliver more oxygen and nutrients to the skin, promoting skin healing and a healthier complexion. This can support the body's natural process of clearing up acne.

Reducing Inflammation: Gua Sha can also help reduce inflammation and stress in the skin, which can prevent new breakouts from forming.

2. Cautions for Acne-Prone Skin

Avoid Active Breakouts: If you have active, inflamed acne (especially cystic acne), avoid using Gua Sha directly over the affected areas. Scraping over open or irritated skin can worsen inflammation and potentially spread bacteria.

Use Light Pressure: Be gentle when using Gua Sha on acne-prone skin. Avoid using heavy pressure on sensitive areas, as this can irritate the skin and trigger new breakouts.

Avoid Infected Areas: Never use Gua Sha over areas with open pimples or pustules to prevent spreading bacteria.

3. Best Products for Acne-Prone Skin

Tea Tree Oil: Tea tree oil has antibacterial properties, making it an excellent choice for acne-prone skin. Pairing Gua Sha with tea tree oil can help fight acne-causing bacteria while soothing the skin.

Niacinamide Serums: Niacinamide helps regulate oil production, reduce redness, and improve skin texture. It can be a great choice to pair with Gua Sha for acne-prone skin.

CREATING A GUA SHA ROUTINE FOR CLEAR, GLOWING SKIN

For Gua Sha to be truly effective in clearing up your complexion and promoting a glowing, radiant skin, consistency is key. Here's how you can structure your routine to get the best results.

1. Start with a Cleanse

Always begin your Gua Sha routine with a thorough cleanse to remove dirt, oil, and impurities. This ensures that the tool doesn't drag on the skin and that products can be absorbed effectively.

2. Hydrate and Apply a Facial Oil or Serum

Apply your favorite hydrating serum or oil to prepare your skin for the tool. This will provide the slip needed to avoid irritation and maximize the benefits of your Gua Sha practice.

3. Perform Gua Sha Strokes

Follow the techniques outlined in previous chapters to perform facial strokes. Focus on areas that need extra attention, such as your jawline, under-eye area, or cheeks.

4. Finish with Moisturizer and Sunscreen

After finishing your Gua Sha routine, apply a moisturizer to lock in the hydration and any active ingredients you've used. If you're doing this in the morning, don't forget to apply sunscreen to protect your skin from UV damage.

5. Frequency

For daily use, focus on light, relaxing strokes to maintain circulation and lymphatic drainage. This helps to maintain a healthy complexion and keeps your skin looking vibrant. For weekly use, you can do deeper, more targeted strokes to treat specific concerns such as puffiness, sagging skin, or uneven texture. Use a little more pressure and focus on areas with tension or wrinkles.

TIPS FOR DAILY VS. WEEKLY GUA SHA SESSIONS

1. Daily Sessions

Purpose: Daily sessions should focus on maintaining skin health, improving circulation, and preventing signs of aging. Keep the pressure light, and focus on gentle gliding strokes that promote lymphatic drainage and circulation.

Time: Spend around 5-10 minutes each day using Gua Sha, depending on your skin's needs.

Frequency: You can perform daily Gua Sha either in the morning or at night, depending on your preference. Many people enjoy using Gua Sha in the morning as a way to de-puff the face and wake up the skin.

2. Weekly Sessions

Purpose: Weekly sessions can be more targeted and intensive, focusing on sculpting the jawline, smoothing fine lines, or addressing muscle tension in the face.

Time: Spend 15-20 minutes on a weekly session to ensure you cover all the target areas, using deeper pressure and more specific techniques.

Frequency: Once a week, or twice if you want to target certain problem areas more intensely.

CHAPTER FIVE

GUA SHA FOR BODY AND MUSCLE RELIEF

While Gua Sha is commonly associated with facial rejuvenation, its benefits extend far beyond the face. When applied to the body, Gua Sha can be a powerful tool for muscle relief, pain management, cellulite reduction, and overall wellness. In this chapter, we will explore how Gua Sha can be used for muscle tension relief, post-workout recovery, and even specific ailments such as headaches, chronic pain, and cellulite.

HOW GUA SHA CAN RELIEVE MUSCLE TENSION AND PAIN

Gua Sha has long been used in Traditional Chinese Medicine (TCM) as a technique to relieve muscle tension, reduce pain, and improve flexibility. The physical benefits of Gua Sha on the body can be particularly helpful for those who suffer from tight muscles, stiffness, or chronic pain.

1. The Mechanism Behind Muscle Relief

Stimulating Blood Flow: Gua Sha stimulates circulation in the tissues, increasing the flow of oxygen-rich blood to areas that are tense or sore. This can help relax the muscles and promote faster recovery.

Breaking Up Muscle Knots: The scraping motion of Gua Sha is effective at breaking up muscle knots (also known as myofascial trigger points). By applying targeted pressure on these knots, Gua Sha helps release tension and restore normal muscle function.

Reducing Inflammation: Chronic pain and muscle tension often lead to inflammation in the affected areas. Gua Sha helps reduce inflammation by encouraging the removal of metabolic waste products from the muscles and improving the drainage of lymphatic fluid, which decreases swelling and promotes healing.

2. Benefits for General Muscle Tension

Gua Sha can be used to alleviate muscle tension caused by a variety of factors, such as stress, poor posture, overuse, or sedentary lifestyles.

Regular use of Gua Sha on tense areas can help prevent the buildup of muscle stiffness, improving overall flexibility and reducing the risk of injury.

APPLYING GUA SHA ON THE NECK, SHOULDERS, AND BACK

The neck, shoulders, and back are common areas of tension due to the stress we carry or from poor posture. Gua Sha is especially effective in releasing this tension, promoting relaxation, and improving mobility in these regions.

1. Neck Relief

Common Issues: Many people suffer from neck stiffness or tension due to long hours of sitting, looking down at devices, or sleeping in awkward positions.

Technique: Using the Gua Sha tool, gently glide from the base of the skull down the sides of the neck to the shoulders. Apply light to moderate pressure, being mindful of sensitive areas. Repeat this motion several times to help relieve tightness.

Focus Areas: Target areas where you feel tension, such as the trapezius muscles at the top of the shoulders or the levator scapulae along the sides of the neck.

2. Shoulder and Upper Back

Common Issues: The shoulders and upper back are also prime areas for muscle tension, especially for those who sit at desks for long periods or engage in repetitive activities.

Technique: Use the tool to glide gently across the shoulder blades and the upper back. Focus on areas where tension is felt, such as along the shoulder girdle or the rhomboid muscles between the shoulder blades. This technique helps release tight muscles, promote blood flow, and reduce pain.

Pressure and Direction: When using Gua Sha on the back and shoulders, begin with gentle pressure and increase it as needed. Always scrape in the direction of muscle fibers to avoid injury and to promote effective muscle relaxation.

3. Lower Back and Spine

Technique: While the spine should be avoided directly, you can use Gua Sha along the paraspinal muscles (the muscles alongside the spine) to help relieve back pain. Glide the tool along these muscles, applying gentle but firm pressure.

Caution: Be careful when using Gua Sha on the lower back, as this area is particularly sensitive. It's important to avoid scraping directly on the spine and to focus on the muscles surrounding it.

GUA SHA FOR CELLULITE REDUCTION AND BODY CONTOURING

In addition to its benefits for muscle relief, Gua Sha has become increasingly popular as a tool for body contouring and cellulite reduction. The technique promotes circulation, improves lymphatic drainage, and helps break down fat deposits beneath the skin.

1. How Gua Sha Helps Reduce Cellulite

Improving Circulation: The scraping action of Gua Sha boosts blood circulation, which helps break down the fat cells that contribute to the appearance of cellulite. As circulation increases, the skin becomes firmer, and the dimples and lumps caused by cellulite begin to smooth out.

Lymphatic Drainage: Gua Sha also stimulates the lymphatic system, encouraging the elimination of toxins and waste products that may contribute to the development of cellulite. This helps reduce fluid retention, which can exacerbate the appearance of dimpled skin.

Targeted Areas: Focus on areas prone to cellulite, such as the thighs, buttocks, and abdomen. Regular Gua Sha sessions can gradually improve the skin's texture and promote smoother, firmer skin.

2. Body Contouring

Lifting and Toning: Gua Sha is also effective for general body contouring. The tool can be used to tone and lift areas that may have lost firmness, such as the inner thighs, upper arms, or abdomen. By applying deep, upward strokes, you can help firm and tighten the skin, promoting a more sculpted appearance.

USING GUA SHA FOR POST-WORKOUT RECOVERY

After a workout, your muscles may feel sore, tight, or fatigued due to the stress placed on them during physical activity. Gua Sha can help speed up recovery by promoting muscle relaxation, reducing soreness, and improving flexibility.

1. How Gua Sha Supports Recovery

Easing Muscle Soreness: After intense exercise, you may experience delayed-onset muscle soreness (DOMS). Gua Sha can help alleviate this discomfort by improving circulation and encouraging the removal of lactic acid and other metabolic waste products from the muscles.

Reducing Inflammation: Gua Sha helps reduce post-workout inflammation by encouraging blood flow to the muscles and promoting the drainage of excess fluids. This can help speed up the healing process and reduce the risk of injury.

2. Post-Workout Routine

After your workout, apply a soothing balm or muscle oil that contains ingredients like arnica, menthol, or eucalyptus to help relax your muscles further. Use the Gua Sha tool gently on the muscles that were most engaged in the workout. Focus on areas like the thighs, calves, lower back, or arms, using long, sweeping strokes to encourage blood flow and relaxation.

ADDRESSING SPECIFIC AILMENTS: HEADACHES, MIGRAINES, AND CHRONIC PAIN

Gua Sha can also be used to address specific ailments that often involve chronic pain or tension, such as headaches, migraines, and muscle pain.

1. Gua Sha for Headaches and Migraines

Technique: Use the Gua Sha tool to gently massage the neck and shoulder area, as tension in these areas is often a trigger for headaches. Begin at the base of the skull and move downward toward the shoulders, applying light pressure and gliding the tool along the muscles of the neck and upper back.

Acupressure Points: Gua Sha can also be used to target acupressure points associated with headache relief, such as the area between the eyebrows or the temples. Lightly apply the tool in circular motions on these points to help release tension and alleviate headache symptoms.

2. Gua Sha for Chronic Pain Relief

Technique: For conditions like chronic back pain, fibromyalgia, or arthritis, use Gua Sha to target the muscles and soft tissues surrounding the painful areas. Glide the tool gently across the affected regions, focusing on muscle groups that are tight or inflamed.

Frequency: Regular Gua Sha sessions can be beneficial for chronic pain management, helping to reduce inflammation, improve flexibility, and promote overall healing.

3. Caution and Consultation

Always consult with a healthcare professional before using Gua Sha for chronic conditions or severe pain, especially if you have injuries or conditions like arthritis, fibromyalgia, or spinal issues. Gua Sha should be used as a complementary treatment, not a substitute for medical care.

CHAPTER SIX

TROUBLESHOOTING GUA SHA TECHNIQUES

While Gua Sha is a safe and effective technique when used correctly, like any new practice, it can come with a learning curve. If you're new to Gua Sha, you may encounter a few bumps along the way, such as redness, bruising, or uneven results. This chapter will guide you on how to troubleshoot common issues that may arise during your Gua Sha practice and provide tips on how to fix them. We'll also discuss when it's necessary to stop and seek professional advice to ensure you're practicing Gua Sha safely and effectively.

WHAT TO DO IF YOU EXPERIENCE REDNESS OR BRUISING

Redness and bruising are common side effects of Gua Sha, especially if you apply too much pressure or use the tool too aggressively. While these effects are typically harmless and usually fade within a few hours or days, they can be concerning if you're not familiar with the process.

1. Understanding Redness and Bruising

Redness: Gua Sha can cause temporary redness as it stimulates blood circulation and promotes the release of stagnated blood and energy (Qi) under the skin. This is a sign that blood flow has increased, and it's typically harmless.

Bruising: Bruising (or "Sha") occurs when there is deeper stagnation or when too much pressure is applied. In Traditional Chinese Medicine, this bruising is considered a release of trapped toxins or blood, but it's important to use caution to avoid excessive marks or pain.

2. What to Do If You Experience Redness or Bruising

Decrease Pressure: If you notice redness or bruising, check that you're not applying too much pressure. Gua Sha should feel like a gentle scraping motion, not an aggressive scraping or digging into the skin.

Adjust Technique: Reduce the intensity of your strokes, especially if you notice bruising forming quickly. Use lighter pressure, particularly over more delicate areas like the under-eye region or thin skin on the neck.

Massage in Short Strokes: Instead of long, continuous strokes, use shorter, gentler strokes. This helps avoid concentrating pressure in one spot for too long.

Allow Time for Healing: If bruising does occur, don't be alarmed. Gua Sha marks typically heal within a few days, but if you want to reduce bruising, apply a cold compress after your session or use healing oils like arnica to support the healing process.

Rest Between Sessions: If bruising persists, consider taking a break from your Gua Sha practice to let your skin fully recover before resuming.

HOW TO ADJUST PRESSURE FOR SENSITIVE SKIN

If you have sensitive skin or are prone to irritation, it's essential to adjust your Gua Sha technique to avoid discomfort or damage. While Gua Sha is generally safe for all skin types, those with delicate skin or underlying skin conditions need to be more mindful of pressure and stroke techniques.

1. Use Gentle Pressure

For sensitive skin, always start with the lightest possible pressure. The tool should glide smoothly without digging into the skin. If you feel resistance or pain, reduce the pressure further.

Light and Slow: Move the tool slowly and steadily. Fast, aggressive movements can irritate the skin and trigger redness or bruising. Slow and controlled strokes promote relaxation and circulation without causing harm.

2. Stick to the Right Tools

Choose a softer Gua Sha tool made from materials like rose quartz or jade. These stones are generally gentler on the skin compared to harder materials like bamboo or horn, which can feel too rough on delicate skin.

Smaller Tools: If you're concerned about pressure, use a smaller Gua Sha tool designed for delicate areas. These tools give you more control and help target specific areas without excess pressure.

3. Avoid Sensitive Areas

Be cautious when using Gua Sha on broken skin, acne, or areas with rosacea. These regions can be more prone to irritation, and the pressure might cause further damage. You can still enjoy the benefits of Gua Sha on other parts of the body, such as the neck and shoulders, while avoiding these sensitive areas.

4. Hydrate and Protect the Skin

Always apply a good layer of moisturizer, serum, or oil before using Gua Sha to ensure your skin is properly hydrated. Dry skin is more susceptible to irritation and could lead to more noticeable redness or irritation. After your session, apply a calming lotion or oil (such as aloe vera, lavender, or chamomile) to soothe the skin.

COMMON MISTAKES TO AVOID IN GUA SHA APPLICATION

Even with the best intentions, it's easy to make a few common mistakes when learning Gua Sha. Here are some errors to be aware of and how to avoid them.

1. Using Too Much Pressure

One of the most common mistakes is applying too much pressure, which can lead to redness, bruising, or irritation. The key is to use enough pressure to create a therapeutic effect without causing harm.

How to Avoid: Start with light pressure and gradually increase if necessary. Gua Sha should feel like a soothing, relaxing massage, not painful or uncomfortable.

2. Scraping in the Wrong Direction

Gua Sha strokes should always be performed in specific directions to enhance their therapeutic benefits. For the face, you want to scrape upward and outward to lift and tone the skin. For the body, strokes should follow the direction of lymphatic flow, which typically moves toward the heart.

How to Avoid: Be mindful of the direction of your strokes. On the face, avoid dragging the tool downward as this can encourage sagging. On the body, follow the natural flow of the lymphatic system to promote detoxification.

3. Not Using Enough Product

Gua Sha requires the use of facial oils, serums, or moisturizers to allow the tool to glide smoothly across the skin. Using Gua Sha without enough product can cause dragging, which can irritate the skin.

How to Avoid: Always apply a generous amount of your chosen serum or oil before beginning your session. The product should give the tool sufficient slip to glide smoothly.

4. Not Cleaning Your Tool

A common but easily avoidable mistake is failing to clean your Gua Sha tool. Over time, oils, dirt, and bacteria can build up on the surface of the tool, which can lead to skin irritation or breakouts.

How to Avoid: Clean your Gua Sha tool after each use with warm water and mild soap or antibacterial wipes. Make sure it's completely dry before storing it.

HOW TO FIX UNEVEN RESULTS OR MISSED AREAS

Sometimes, Gua Sha results may seem uneven or you may realize that you missed some spots, particularly when you're still learning the techniques.

1. Uneven Results

If one side of your face or body appears more lifted than the other, it could be due to uneven pressure or technique during your session.

How to Fix: If you notice uneven results, try adjusting the pressure on the side that is less responsive. Repeat the strokes for a few extra minutes on the side that needs more attention. Make sure to use consistent pressure on both sides during each session.

2. Missed Areas

It's easy to miss certain spots when using Gua Sha, especially on large areas like the back or body.

How to Fix: After completing your Gua Sha routine, take a moment to inspect your skin and check for any areas that may have been missed. Gently apply the tool to those areas with light pressure, using upward or outward strokes as needed.

WHEN TO STOP AND SEEK PROFESSIONAL ADVICE

While Gua Sha is generally safe, there are times when it's necessary to stop and seek professional advice, particularly if you encounter issues that don't resolve after adjusting your technique.

1. Persistent Pain or Discomfort

If you experience persistent pain, discomfort, or sharp sensations during or after your Gua Sha session, stop immediately and reassess your technique. This could indicate that you're using too much pressure or applying the tool incorrectly.

When to Seek Professional Help: If the discomfort continues or worsens, consult with a dermatologist, licensed practitioner, or healthcare provider.

2. Pre-existing Skin Conditions

If you have skin conditions like eczema, psoriasis, or broken skin, Gua Sha might irritate these conditions further.

When to Seek Professional Help: If you're unsure whether Gua Sha is suitable for your skin, it's best to consult with a healthcare professional or dermatologist before continuing.

3. Unresolved Bruising or Redness

If bruising or redness doesn't fade within a few days, or if it becomes more severe, stop using the tool and seek medical advice. Persistent bruising could indicate that you are applying excessive pressure or that there is an underlying health concern.

CHAPTER SEVEN

ADVANCED GUA SHA TECHNIQUES

As you become more comfortable with the basics of Gua Sha, it's time to explore advanced techniques that can enhance your results, deepen your understanding of the practice, and address specific areas of concern more effectively. In this chapter, we'll focus on advanced Gua Sha methods for neck and décolletage toning, facial acupressure, sculpting and contouring, and integrating Gua Sha into your holistic wellness routine. We'll also discuss how to customize your Gua Sha practice based on your unique skin type and beauty goals.

MASTERING GUA SHA FOR NECK AND DÉCOLLETAGE TONING

The neck and décolletage (upper chest) are areas that often show signs of aging, such as sagging skin, fine lines, and wrinkles, and they are commonly neglected during skincare routines. Gua Sha is a powerful tool for toning these areas, reducing tension, and boosting circulation, helping to restore a youthful appearance.

1. Why Focus on the Neck and Décolletage?

Delicate Skin: The skin on the neck and chest is thinner and more delicate, making it prone to sagging, wrinkles, and environmental damage.

Tension Release: These areas can accumulate tension, especially for those who spend long hours looking down at devices, which contributes to neck stiffness and the development of tech neck.

Enhanced Blood Flow: Gua Sha promotes circulation, which can help reduce the appearance of wrinkles, improve skin tone, and encourage cell turnover.

2. Technique for Neck Toning

Step 1: Start at the Jawline: Begin by placing the Gua Sha tool at the jawline and gently scrape down toward the collarbones. Use light pressure, following the natural contours of the neck.

Step 2: Move Along the Neck: Work your way down the sides of the neck, scraping in upward motions to promote lifting. For more defined jawline contours, make sure to apply gentle pressure around the mandible and work in an upward direction.

Step 3: Focus on the Décolletage: To target the décolletage, use long, sweeping strokes starting from the top of the chest near the clavicle and glide the tool toward the shoulders. This will improve lymphatic drainage, reduce puffiness, and promote firmer skin.

3. Pro Tips

Avoid the Thyroid Area: Be mindful to avoid the thyroid area in the center of the neck, as this area is particularly sensitive.

Frequency: Practice Gua Sha on the neck and décolletage 2-3 times per week for noticeable toning and lifting effects.

COMBINING GUA SHA WITH FACIAL ACUPRESSURE FOR DEEPER HEALING

Combining Gua Sha with facial acupressure can elevate the healing and rejuvenating benefits of your practice. Acupressure involves applying targeted pressure to specific points on the face and body to stimulate the flow of energy, or Qi, promote relaxation, and encourage healing.

1. How Facial Acupressure Enhances Gua Sha

Deepens Relaxation: Acupressure points help reduce stress, calm the nervous system, and support overall wellness.

Improves Circulation: Acupressure helps to open up blocked energy pathways, increasing blood flow to the face, which supports skin health, enhances radiance, and promotes detoxification.

Addresses Specific Concerns: By targeting acupressure points related to specific areas of concern (such as acne, puffiness, or wrinkles), you can address both physical and energetic imbalances.

2. Key Acupressure Points for the Face

Here are some common facial acupressure points that can be combined with Gua Sha to enhance the effects:

Third Eye Point (Yintang): Located between the eyebrows, this point is used to relieve stress, headaches, and promote relaxation. Apply gentle pressure here before starting your Gua Sha routine.

Temple Points: At the temples, this area helps relieve tension, alleviate headaches, and improve overall circulation to the face.

Jaw Points (Stomach 7): Located just below the cheekbones, these points help relieve jaw tension and can help with facial contouring.

Chin Point (Ren 24): This point is found at the center of the chin and is believed to help with fluid retention and to support a lifted appearance.

3. Technique

Before starting your Gua Sha routine, massage these acupressure points with gentle circular motions for 1-2 minutes using your fingertips. Once you've activated these points, follow with your Gua Sha strokes on the face, working in an upward and outward direction. This combination enhances the blood flow to the skin, promotes a healthier complexion, and deepens relaxation.

GUA SHA FOR SCULPTING AND CONTOURING THE FACE

One of the most popular uses of Gua Sha is for facial sculpting and contouring. With consistent practice, Gua Sha can help define your cheekbones, jawline, and eyebrows, while also lifting and firming the skin.

1. Sculpting the Jawline

Step 1: Place the Gua Sha tool under your jawline, at the center of the chin.

Step 2: Scrape the tool outward along the jawline toward the ears, applying moderate pressure. This helps define the jawline and reduce the appearance of a double chin.

Pro Tip: For added contouring, use a V-shaped Gua Sha tool for better precision along the jawline.

2. Lifting the Cheeks

Step 1: Begin at the sides of your nose and gently scrape upwards toward the temples.

Step 2: Repeat this motion several times to lift the cheekbones and promote a more youthful appearance.

Pro Tip: Focus on the area just beneath the cheekbones to enhance the appearance of fullness and lift.

3. Defining the Eyebrows

Step 1: Place the tool at the bridge of the nose and gently glide upwards towards the eyebrows.

Step 2: Continue scraping along the brow bone to the temples to lift and define the eyebrows.

Pro Tip: To open the eyes and reduce puffiness, concentrate on the area around the under-eye socket.

4. Frequency

For visible sculpting and contouring, practice these techniques 3-4 times a week. Over time, you should notice more definition in the jawline, cheeks, and overall facial structure.

INCORPORATING GUA SHA INTO YOUR HOLISTIC WELLNESS ROUTINE

Gua Sha is not just a skincare technique it's an important part of a holistic wellness approach that incorporates physical, emotional, and energetic healing. By integrating Gua Sha into your overall wellness routine, you can achieve deeper relaxation, detoxification, and balance.

1. Mindful Practice

Take a moment to center yourself before starting your Gua Sha routine. Deep breathing or meditation can help calm the mind and prepare your body for the healing process.

Use Gua Sha as an opportunity to release stress and negative energy. Visualize the scraping motion as a way to release stagnation in both your body and mind.

2. Holistic Wellness Benefits

Stress Relief: By combining Gua Sha with acupressure and deep breathing, you activate the body's parasympathetic nervous system, helping to reduce stress and promote relaxation.

Improved Sleep: Gua Sha can be a part of your bedtime routine to help calm the mind and relieve tension, potentially improving your sleep quality.

Emotional Balance: Gua Sha can help release emotional blockages, reduce anxiety, and promote a sense of calm and clarity.

3. Supporting Detoxification

Gua Sha can assist in detoxifying the skin and body by improving lymphatic drainage and circulation. After your session, consider drinking water or herbal teas that support detoxification to aid in the elimination of toxins.

CUSTOMIZING YOUR GUA SHA PRACTICE BASED ON SKIN TYPE AND GOALS

Everyone's skin is unique, and tailoring your Gua Sha practice to your skin type and beauty goals will optimize the benefits. Here's how to customize your routine based on your individual needs.

1. Dry or Dehydrated Skin

Use Rich Oils: Choose moisturizing oils or serums that are rich in hydrating ingredients, such as hyaluronic acid, squalane, or jojoba oil.

Gentle Pressure: Focus on using gentle pressure to avoid any irritation to your skin. Be sure to apply enough product to keep the tool gliding smoothly.

2. Oily or Acne-Prone Skin

Non-comedogenic Products: Opt for lightweight, oil-free products that won't clog pores. Look for products containing niacinamide, salicylic acid, or tea tree oil to help balance oil production.

Avoid Active Acne Areas: If you have active breakouts, avoid directly scraping over acne lesions to prevent irritation. Instead, focus on areas with congestion or tension.

3. Mature Skin

Firming Products: For mature skin, use firming serums that contain ingredients like retinol, **peptides

CHAPTER EIGHT

CREATING A GUA SHA ROUTINE FOR MAXIMUM BENEFITS

Developing a consistent Gua Sha routine is key to unlocking its full potential and achieving the most noticeable results. Whether you're aiming to enhance your skin's appearance, relieve muscle tension, or promote overall wellness, establishing the right frequency, timing, and technique can make a big difference. In this chapter, we'll guide you on how to create a personalized Gua Sha routine, including when to perform it (morning or evening), how often to practice, how to structure your weekly sessions, and how to pair it with other skincare and wellness practices for optimal results. Additionally, we'll discuss how to track your progress and celebrate your milestones.

MORNING VS. EVENING GUA SHA: WHICH WORKS BEST FOR YOU?

The timing of your Gua Sha sessions can influence your results, as both morning and evening practices offer unique benefits. The key is to align your routine with your skin's needs, energy levels, and lifestyle.

1. Morning Gua Sha: Energize and Refresh

Boosts Circulation: Starting your day with Gua Sha helps stimulate blood flow, oxygenate the skin, and provide a natural glow. It also supports lymphatic drainage, helping to reduce puffiness and swelling, particularly around the eyes and face.

Energizing: Gua Sha in the morning can help wake you up and give you a sense of refreshment. The act of scraping stimulates the body and the face, which can enhance alertness and energy levels.

Preps for the Day: By incorporating Gua Sha in the morning, you're effectively priming your skin for makeup application. The stimulation of circulation helps products absorb more effectively and creates a smoother base.

When to Use Gua Sha in the Morning:

Time: Ideally, perform Gua Sha after your morning skincare routine, just before applying sunscreen and makeup. This helps the products penetrate better and boosts the effectiveness of your other skincare steps.

Focus: Prioritize areas that experience puffiness, like the under-eye area, the jawline, and the forehead.

2. Evening Gua Sha: Relax and Recover

Stress Relief: Evening Gua Sha helps unwind from the day's tension, especially in areas like the neck, shoulders, and jaw. It is ideal for reducing muscle tightness, headaches, or the effects of stress.

Promotes Relaxation: This is a great time to combine Gua Sha with facial acupressure or meditation to relax the mind and body before bed.

Enhances Skin Repair: Nighttime is when your skin is most receptive to repair. By using Gua Sha in the evening, you're boosting circulation and lymphatic drainage, which aids in the body's natural detox processes and supports skin renewal overnight.

When to Use Gua Sha in the Evening:

Time: Perform your Gua Sha routine after your evening skincare routine, just before going to bed. It can be a calming ritual to prepare your skin for a restorative sleep.

Focus: Concentrate on releasing tension in the neck, jaw, and shoulders. If you're looking for facial sculpting, spend more time on the jawline, cheeks, and forehead.

Which One Works Best for You?

If you're someone who wakes up feeling sluggish, starting the day with Gua Sha might be your best option to energize both body and face. If you experience stress or muscle tension, an evening routine can help relieve that discomfort and encourage relaxation before sleep.

HOW OFTEN SHOULD YOU PRACTICE GUA SHA FOR OPTIMAL RESULTS?

The frequency of your Gua Sha sessions will depend on your skin's sensitivity, your personal goals, and how much time you have to dedicate to the practice. Overuse or improper technique can lead to irritation, so it's important to find a balanced routine.

1. Daily Gua Sha

Best for: Those seeking to maintain glowing, youthful skin and improve circulation. A gentle, daily practice can also support lymphatic drainage and reduce puffiness.

Time: 5–10 minutes per session.

Techniques: Stick to lighter pressure and shorter strokes, especially if you're just starting. Focus on the face, with emphasis on areas like the jawline, forehead, and under-eye area.

2. 3–4 Times a Week

Best for: Those looking to enhance contouring, relieve muscle tension, or target specific skin concerns such as sagging, fine lines, or acne. This frequency provides a balance between achieving results and allowing your skin time to recover.

Time: 10–15 minutes per session.

Techniques: Use moderate pressure with longer, more deliberate strokes. Include both facial and body Gua Sha to address concerns like neck tension or cellulite.

3. Weekly Gua Sha

Best for: Beginners or those with sensitive skin. Less frequent sessions allow your skin time to adjust to the practice without risk of bruising or irritation.

Time: 15–20 minutes per session.

Techniques: Focus on specific areas you want to treat, and use gentle pressure. You can incorporate deeper techniques such as facial acupressure or muscle relief on the body.

How to Decide Frequency:

Sensitive Skin: Start with 2–3 times a week and increase as your skin gets used to the practice.

Goal-Oriented: If your goal is facial sculpting or muscle relief, practicing more frequently (3–4 times a week) may deliver faster results.

STRUCTURING YOUR WEEKLY GUA SHA ROUTINE

To make the most of your Gua Sha sessions, structure your weekly practice based on your skin's needs and wellness goals. Here's a sample weekly schedule that incorporates a variety of Gua Sha techniques:

1. Monday: Lymphatic Drainage and Facial Lifting

Focus: Promote circulation and reduce puffiness. Spend time on the jawline, cheeks, and under-eye area.

Techniques: Light pressure, upward strokes. Use a cooling, hydrating serum or oil for smooth glide.

Benefit: Start the week with a refreshed, glowing complexion.

2. Tuesday: Neck and Décolletage Toning

Focus: Sculpt and firm the neck and chest area, which are prone to sagging and fine lines.

Techniques: Long, upward strokes on the neck and chest, using moderate pressure.

Benefit: Toned and lifted appearance, with reduced tension.

3. Wednesday: Muscle Tension Relief (Body Gua Sha)

Focus: Target the neck, shoulders, and upper back for muscle relaxation. This is particularly beneficial for those with desk jobs or tension headaches.

Techniques: Stronger pressure and longer strokes. Focus on the shoulders, neck, and upper back to relieve tightness.

Benefit: Release physical stress, improve posture, and reduce discomfort.

4. Thursday: Acupressure and Facial Relaxation

Focus: Combine facial acupressure with light Gua Sha strokes to enhance relaxation and reduce stress.

Techniques: Apply gentle pressure to acupressure points, followed by gentle Gua Sha strokes.

Benefit: Enhanced relaxation, improved skin tone, and reduced signs of stress.

5. Friday: Sculpting and Contouring

Focus: Sculpt the jawline, cheekbones, and forehead for a more contoured appearance.

Techniques: Use more pressure and focus on defined strokes to enhance contouring and lift.

Benefit: Sharper, more sculpted facial features.

6. Saturday: Full Body Gua Sha (Optional)

Focus: Incorporate full-body Gua Sha for cellulite reduction, muscle relief, and detoxification.

Techniques: Long strokes over thighs, arms, and back to promote detox and smooth skin texture.

Benefit: Relaxed muscles, improved lymphatic drainage, and smooth skin.

7. Sunday: Rest and Recovery

Focus: Take a break from your regular routine to allow your skin to recover.

Benefit: This rest period gives your skin time to rejuvenate and prepare for the next week's practice.

PAIRING GUA SHA WITH OTHER SKINCARE AND WELLNESS PRACTICES

To maximize the benefits of Gua Sha, consider pairing it with other practices that complement and support your skin's health and overall wellness. Here are a few ideas:

1. Pairing with Skincare

Hydration: Use a hydrating serum or facial oil before your Gua Sha practice to prevent skin dragging. This ensures the tool glides smoothly.

Masks: Apply a nourishing face mask before or after Gua Sha to lock in moisture and support skin repair.

Sunscreen: Always finish your routine with SPF to protect the skin from UV damage, especially if you practice Gua Sha in the morning.

2. Pairing with Wellness Practices

Meditation: Pair Gua Sha with a few minutes of deep breathing or meditation for relaxation.

Yoga: Incorporate Gua Sha after your yoga practice to release muscle tension and promote relaxation.

Herbal Teas: Drink herbal teas that support detoxification, like chamomile or ginger, after your Gua Sha routine to enhance lymphatic drainage and promote

CHAPTER NINE

GUA SHA FOR DIFFERENT SKIN TYPES

Gua Sha is a versatile and adaptive skincare tool, offering benefits to various skin types. However, to ensure you're getting the most out of your practice, it's important to tailor your approach to meet the unique needs of your skin. Whether you have oily, dry, mature, or combination skin, Gua Sha can be used to promote balance, soothe irritation, reduce signs of aging, and more. This chapter will provide guidance on how to customize your Gua Sha routine for each skin type, maximizing its benefits and preventing any potential irritation.

GUA SHA FOR OILY AND ACNE-PRONE SKIN: BEST PRACTICES

For those with oily or acne-prone skin, Gua Sha can be a powerful tool to support balance and enhance circulation. However, it's important to approach it with care to avoid irritation or aggravating existing breakouts.

1. Why Gua Sha Helps Oily and Acne-Prone Skin

Lymphatic Drainage: Gua Sha aids in the removal of toxins and excess fluids, which can contribute to puffiness and breakouts. Improved lymphatic drainage helps prevent blockages in the pores, reducing the frequency and severity of acne.

Improved Circulation: By stimulating blood flow to the face, Gua Sha helps oxygenate the skin, encourage healing, and promote a healthier complexion.

Reduces Stress: Acne can sometimes be exacerbated by stress. The relaxing effect of Gua Sha can help lower stress levels, thus supporting clearer skin.

2. Best Practices for Oily and Acne-Prone Skin

Use Non-Comedogenic Oils: Opt for lightweight, non-comedogenic oils like jojoba oil, grapeseed oil, or tea tree oil. These oils are less likely to clog pores and can provide antibacterial benefits for acne-prone skin.

Avoid Active Breakout Areas: When practicing Gua Sha, avoid applying direct pressure over active acne or inflamed areas to prevent irritation. Instead, focus on other areas of the face, such as the jawline, neck, and forehead, or areas with congestion.

Gentle Pressure: Apply light pressure to avoid aggravating the skin. Overuse of pressure could cause redness or irritation.

Targeting Congestion: Use Gua Sha on areas where clogged pores or blackheads are common, like the nose and chin. This can help break down impurities and promote clearer skin.

3. Frequency

2-3 Times a Week: For oily and acne-prone skin, practice Gua Sha 2–3 times a week to avoid over-stimulation. Gradually increase frequency as your skin becomes accustomed to the technique.

GUA SHA FOR DRY AND SENSITIVE SKIN: HOW TO ADAPT THE TECHNIQUE

Dry and sensitive skin types require a more gentle approach when using Gua Sha. Dry skin tends to be more prone to irritation, flakiness, and redness, while sensitive skin can react to harsher techniques or pressure. Fortunately, with the right adjustments, Gua Sha can work wonders for these skin types.

1. Why Gua Sha Helps Dry and Sensitive Skin

Boosts Hydration: Gua Sha helps stimulate circulation and allows better absorption of moisturizers and hydrating serums, helping to lock in moisture and prevent dehydration.

Gentle Exfoliation: The scraping action of Gua Sha encourages the shedding of dead skin cells, revealing a smoother, softer texture, without the need for harsh exfoliants.

Reduces Puffiness and Inflammation: Gua Sha can help soothe inflamed or irritated skin, reducing redness and promoting lymphatic drainage to alleviate puffiness, especially under the eyes.

2. Best Practices for Dry and Sensitive Skin

Hydrating Oils and Serums: Use a rich, hydrating serum or oil before your Gua Sha practice to ensure smooth gliding and to provide the necessary moisture for dry or sensitive skin. Look for products with hyaluronic acid, squalane, or rosehip oil for extra hydration and nourishment.

Gentle Pressure and Strokes: For dry and sensitive skin, use light pressure and shorter strokes. This will avoid any discomfort or irritation and allow for more control during the practice.

Focus on Lymphatic Drainage: Gua Sha is excellent for supporting lymphatic drainage, which can help reduce puffiness and the appearance of redness, especially around the eyes and cheeks. Focus on lifting motions along the jawline, forehead, and neck.

Avoid Scraping Over Broken Skin: If you have any areas of broken skin, rashes, or severe dryness, it's best to avoid using the Gua Sha tool directly on these areas to prevent further irritation.

3. Frequency

3-4 Times a Week: Sensitive and dry skin should ideally receive Gua Sha treatment 3–4 times a week. This frequency strikes a balance between boosting circulation and providing the skin enough time to rest and heal.

GUA SHA FOR MATURE SKIN: PREVENTING SAGGING AND WRINKLES

Mature skin, often characterized by loss of elasticity, fine lines, and wrinkles, can greatly benefit from Gua Sha's lifting and toning effects. Regular practice can help rejuvenate the skin and encourage a more youthful, firm appearance.

1. Why Gua Sha Helps Mature Skin

Stimulates Collagen Production: Gua Sha helps stimulate collagen and elastin production by promoting circulation, which can help firm and plump the skin over time.

Lifts and Tightens: Gua Sha's scraping motion works as a natural facial sculpting technique, lifting and tightening sagging skin, particularly around the jawline, cheeks, and neck.

Reduces Fine Lines and Wrinkles: By improving circulation and increasing skin's oxygenation, Gua Sha can reduce the appearance of fine lines, making skin appear more youthful and smooth.

2. Best Practices for Mature Skin

Use Firming Oils: Opt for products with peptides, retinol, or Vitamin C, which are known for their anti-aging benefits. These ingredients can help firm, brighten, and reduce the appearance of wrinkles.

Moderate Pressure for Lift: Use moderate pressure and longer strokes to focus on areas prone to sagging, such as the jawline, neck, and cheeks. This will help lift and define these areas while improving skin texture.

Focus on Specific Areas: Pay extra attention to crow's feet, nasolabial folds, and the neck area. These are the common trouble spots where sagging and wrinkles often become more prominent with age.

3. Frequency

4-5 Times a Week: For mature skin, Gua Sha can be used more frequently, up to 4-5 times a week, especially when targeting areas with sagging or fine lines. You may also want to include facial acupressure for deeper rejuvenation.

CUSTOMIZING GUA SHA FOR COMBINATION SKIN

Combination skin typically involves areas of both oily and dry skin, with the T-zone (forehead, nose, chin) being more oily and the cheeks and jawline being drier or more sensitive. For combination skin, the goal is to balance both skin concerns while ensuring you don't aggravate any areas.

1. Why Gua Sha Helps Combination Skin

Balances Oil Production: Gua Sha can help regulate oil production in the T-zone, especially when used with oil-controlling products like niacinamide or salicylic acid.

Hydrates Dry Areas: For drier areas, Gua Sha enhances the absorption of moisturizers and hydrating serums, helping to soothe and replenish moisture without causing oil buildup.

Targets Specific Concerns: By customizing your strokes and technique, Gua Sha can address multiple skin concerns simultaneously whether it's reducing shine, promoting hydration, or sculpting and toning.

2. Best Practices for Combination Skin

Use Tailored Products: Select a serum or oil that works well for both oil-control and hydration. Consider hyaluronic acid for dry areas and niacinamide or salicylic acid for the oily T-zone.

Focus on Targeted Areas: Use Gua Sha to focus on the T-zone to promote lymphatic drainage and reduce excess oil, and apply more nourishing oils or serums to the dry areas (like the cheeks and jawline).

Pressure Adjustments: Apply slightly more pressure to areas that are prone to congestion (like the nose and forehead) and use lighter strokes on the more sensitive, drier areas.

3. Frequency

3-4 Times a Week: Combination skin responds well to a consistent but moderate routine. Use Gua Sha 3–4 times a week, focusing on balancing both hydration and oil control.

THE ROLE OF GUA SHA IN PROMOTING SKIN HEALTH OVER TIME

While Gua Sha offers immediate benefits like improved circulation, relaxation, and reduced puffiness, the true magic happens over time. With consistent practice, Gua Sha can support skin health in a variety of ways, promoting long-term improvements in texture, tone, and appearance.

CHAPTER TEN

THE EMOTIONAL AND PSYCHOLOGICAL BENEFITS OF GUA SHA

While Gua Sha is commonly known for its physical benefits such as improving circulation, reducing puffiness, and relieving muscle tension the practice also offers significant emotional and psychological advantages. When practiced mindfully and incorporated into a regular wellness routine, Gua Sha can be a powerful tool for stress relief, emotional balance, and self-care. This chapter will explore how Gua Sha can enhance your mental and emotional well-being, foster self-love, and help cultivate a deeper connection with yourself.

GUA SHA AS A TOOL FOR STRESS RELIEF AND RELAXATION

In today's fast-paced world, stress and anxiety have become common, affecting not just our mental health but also our physical well-being. Gua Sha can help relieve the physical manifestations of stress, such as tight muscles, tension, and a lack of relaxation, while also supporting a calmer, more centered emotional state.

1. Stress-Relieving Properties

Releases Physical Tension: Stress often manifests in the body as tightness in the shoulders, neck, and jaw. Gua Sha's scraping motion stimulates the fascia (the connective tissue surrounding muscles), helping to release tension and promote relaxation. This release of physical tightness can have a profound effect on your mental and emotional state.

Stimulates the Vagus Nerve: The Vagus nerve is a key component of the parasympathetic nervous system, which helps regulate our relaxation response. By using Gua Sha with gentle pressure, particularly on areas like the neck, shoulders, and jaw, you can stimulate this nerve, activating the body's natural relaxation response and reducing anxiety.

Improves Circulation and Oxygen Flow: Increased blood flow and circulation from Gua Sha support the body's natural detoxification processes and provide a sense of overall well-being. This helps to reduce the physiological effects of stress, like shallow breathing and a racing heart.

2. Relaxation and Mind-Body Connection

A Calming Ritual: Performing Gua Sha can become a meditative and calming ritual in your daily routine. The repetitive motions of scraping the skin with a smooth tool can become deeply soothing, allowing you to unwind and create space for mindfulness.

Slowing Down: The act of taking time for yourself, applying gentle pressure, and focusing on your body during a Gua Sha session can bring a sense of calm and help you connect with your breath. This practice encourages you to slow down, breathe deeply, and be present, helping you disconnect from the stresses of daily life.

MINDFUL GUA SHA: USING THE PRACTICE FOR EMOTIONAL BALANCE

Mindfulness is the practice of being fully present and engaged in the moment, without judgment. When you incorporate mindfulness into your Gua Sha routine, it can help regulate emotions, enhance your self-awareness, and bring a sense of emotional balance and calm.

1. How to Practice Mindful Gua Sha

Set an Intention: Before you begin your Gua Sha session, take a moment to set an intention for the practice. This could be something simple, like "I am relaxing and releasing stress," or more specific, such as "I am letting go of tension in my neck and shoulders." Setting an intention helps ground you and gives your practice direction.

Breathing and Focus: As you apply the tool to your face or body, focus on your breath. Take slow, deep breaths as you glide the Gua Sha tool over your skin. Pay attention to how your body feels and notice any areas that feel tight or tense. Breathe into those areas, and imagine releasing any emotional weight or stress with each exhale.

Listen to Your Body: Mindful Gua Sha involves tuning into your body's signals. If you feel discomfort or tension, adjust your pressure or focus on a different area. Don't rush the practice allow yourself to enjoy the sensation of the tool gliding over your skin, the heat it generates, and the calming rhythm it creates.

2. Emotional Healing Through Gua Sha

Releasing Stored Emotions: Our bodies often store emotional tension, particularly in areas such as the shoulders, jaw, and chest. As you move the Gua Sha tool over these areas, you may experience an emotional release a sense of lightness or even tears. This release is part of the healing process, as Gua Sha can help unblock energy that has been stored physically in the body.

Creating Emotional Balance: Regularly practicing mindful Gua Sha can support emotional stability. By practicing self-care and creating time to focus on yourself, you encourage emotional balance and help regulate mood fluctuations. The calming effects of Gua Sha help you approach challenges with a clearer, calmer mind.

HOW GUA SHA ENHANCES YOUR SELF-CARE ROUTINE

Self-care is about nurturing your body, mind, and spirit, and Gua Sha can be a significant addition to your wellness routine. By integrating Gua Sha into your daily or weekly rituals, you can cultivate a sense of peace, well-being, and self-love.

1. A Holistic Practice

Gua Sha is not just about external beauty it's about taking time for yourself and nurturing your physical and emotional health. When you engage in this practice, you are actively creating space for relaxation, balance, and healing. It's a holistic form of self-care that supports both your mental and physical health.

2. Ritualizing Your Gua Sha Practice

Evening Routine: After a long day, Gua Sha can be a soothing way to unwind. Pair your evening Gua Sha practice with calming activities like a warm bath, drinking herbal tea, or listening to relaxing music to create a deeply restorative ritual.

Morning Routine: If you prefer starting your day with Gua Sha, it can help refresh and awaken your skin, as well as invigorate your mind. It sets the tone for the day, providing a moment of mindfulness and self-nourishment.

Weekly Ritual: If you find daily practice too time-consuming, consider incorporating Gua Sha into a weekly self-care ritual. Set aside a specific time each week for a longer session, allowing yourself to fully relax and indulge in this rejuvenating practice.

CULTIVATING SELF-LOVE AND CONFIDENCE THROUGH GUA SHA

Gua Sha is not just a tool for physical beauty it can also be a transformative practice for cultivating self-love and boosting confidence. The act of caring for your body and dedicating time to yourself can improve how you view yourself, increase self-esteem, and reinforce positive feelings about your appearance and your worth.

1. Reaffirming Your Worth

Taking the time to perform a Gua Sha routine is an act of self-care and self-respect. By prioritizing your well-being and making self-care a non-negotiable part of your routine, you reinforce the idea that you deserve to feel good, look good, and be healthy. This helps to shift your mindset, fostering a greater sense of self-worth and confidence.

2. Building Confidence Through Self-Care

Aesthetic Benefits: While the physical benefits of Gua Sha, such as improved skin tone, reduction in puffiness, and facial sculpting, are noticeable, the confidence that comes from taking care of yourself is even more powerful. When you feel good in your skin, your confidence naturally grows.

Self-Acceptance: Gua Sha encourages you to accept and embrace your body as it is, nurturing it with love and care. This act of self-nurturing can shift your perception of yourself, reinforcing the idea that you are worthy of time, attention, and love.

THE THERAPEUTIC EFFECTS OF REGULAR GUA SHA SESSIONS

When practiced regularly, Gua Sha can have therapeutic effects on both the body and mind, acting as a form of holistic therapy that promotes emotional healing, mental clarity, and overall well-being.

1. Emotional Detox

Regular Gua Sha practice helps to release both physical and emotional blockages, allowing for emotional detoxification. As tension and stress are released, you create space for new, positive energy, leading to a more peaceful and balanced emotional state.

2. Increased Resilience

The therapeutic benefits of Gua Sha can enhance emotional resilience over time. By making self-care a consistent part of your routine, you cultivate the ability to face life's challenges with greater calm and poise. This enhances your emotional stamina, helping you navigate stress, uncertainty, and difficult emotions more effectively.

3. Better Sleep and Relaxation

The relaxation benefits of Gua Sha can extend to better sleep, as it helps release tension and promote relaxation before bed. A soothing Gua Sha session can be the perfect way to wind down and prepare for restful, restorative sleep.

CONCLUSION

EMBRACING THE GUA SHA JOURNEY

As you conclude this exploration of Gua Sha, it's important to recognize that this practice is not just a beauty or wellness trend it's a timeless tool that offers profound benefits for your body, mind, and spirit. Whether you are just beginning or have become an experienced practitioner, Gua Sha provides an opportunity to connect with your body in a meaningful and intentional way. It is a ritual of self-care, a journey of self-love, and a pathway to long-term wellness. Let's take a moment to celebrate your Gua Sha journey and reflect on how you can maintain and integrate the benefits of this practice into your daily life.

CELEBRATING YOUR GUA SHA JOURNEY: FROM BEGINNER TO EXPERT

The journey from a beginner to an expert in Gua Sha is one of gradual discovery, learning, and growth. In the beginning, you may have felt unsure about how to use the tool or worried about getting the technique right. But over time, as you practiced and observed the benefits, you began to gain confidence in your abilities and understanding. Whether you've just started your Gua Sha routine or have been practicing for a while, each session is an opportunity to refine your technique, discover new benefits, and further deepen your connection with yourself.

1. A Gradual Mastery Process: Mastery of Gua Sha comes with time and consistency. At first, you may focus on learning the basic strokes, experimenting with different tools, and figuring out the right pressure and technique. As you continue practicing, you'll find that the motions become second nature, and your skill level improves. This sense of mastery is incredibly rewarding, not just for the physical results you see, but also for the mindfulness and emotional benefits you experience.

2. From Beginner to Expert: Trusting Your Intuition Over time, you'll start to trust your intuition more when practicing Gua Sha. You'll know which areas of your body or face need more attention and which require gentler strokes. Your connection with your body will deepen, allowing you to personalize your sessions to meet your ever-changing needs. The journey toward expertise is as much about listening to your body as it is about technique.

STAYING CONSISTENT: HOW TO MAINTAIN THE BENEFITS OF GUA SHA

To experience the full benefits of Gua Sha, consistency is key. Like any practice, the more regularly you engage with it, the more pronounced the results. Whether you choose to practice daily, several times a week, or as part of a weekly ritual, staying consistent will help you maintain the positive effects on your skin, muscles, and overall sense of well-being.

1. Creating a Sustainable Routine: While consistency is important, it's also essential to make your Gua Sha practice fit seamlessly into your lifestyle. Whether it's part of your morning skincare routine or your evening wind-down ritual, find a time that works for you. Setting aside just 5-10 minutes a day can yield lasting benefits, and over time, Gua Sha will become a cherished ritual in your self-care routine.

2. Adapting to Your Needs: Your needs may evolve over time, whether due to changes in your skin, emotional state, or physical health. As you continue with your Gua

Sha practice, be open to adapting your routine. For instance, you may find that some areas need more attention during stressful periods or that your skin requires extra hydration in the winter months. Being flexible and responsive to your body's signals will allow you to get the most out of your Gua Sha practice.

FINAL THOUGHTS ON INTEGRATING GUA SHA INTO YOUR DAILY LIFE

Integrating Gua Sha into your daily life is not just about the immediate benefits you see glowing skin, reduced puffiness, or alleviated tension it's about cultivating a holistic practice that nourishes your body and soul. The practice of Gua Sha encourages mindfulness, self-care, and personal connection, creating space for relaxation, healing, and growth. As you continue your Gua Sha journey, remember that it is a deeply personal practice that will evolve with you over time.

1. Make It a Holistic Part of Your Wellness As you integrate Gua Sha into your daily life, consider how it fits into your broader wellness routine. Pairing it with other

practices such as yoga, meditation, or healthy eating can enhance its benefits and contribute to a balanced, mindful lifestyle. Gua Sha is a tool that complements a holistic approach to health and beauty supporting both your external appearance and internal well-being.

2. Be Gentle with Yourself Self-care is about treating yourself with kindness and compassion, and Gua Sha can be a reminder to slow down and prioritize your own well-being. As you continue to practice, remember that there is no "perfect" way to do Gua Sha what matters most is that you are taking time to nurture your body, relax your mind, and show yourself the love you deserve.

EMBRACING GUA SHA FOR LONG-TERM BEAUTY AND WELLNESS

Incorporating Gua Sha into your life is a powerful choice that can have lasting benefits, not just for your physical appearance, but for your emotional and mental health. Whether you're seeking to reduce signs of aging, relieve muscle tension, or simply find a moment of peace in a busy day, Gua Sha is a tool that offers long-term value.

The deeper you engage with it, the more you'll find that it's not just about enhancing your outer beauty, but cultivating a sense of well-being that permeates all areas of your life.

1. Gua Sha as a Long-Term Investment As you continue your practice, view Gua Sha as an investment in your long-term beauty and wellness. It's a practice that doesn't just offer immediate results, but also promotes lasting health and vitality. Over time, you'll notice cumulative benefits whether in the way your skin looks, how your body feels, or how you feel emotionally and mentally.

2. A Lifelong Wellness Tool Gua Sha is a timeless practice that has been passed down for generations in traditional healing systems. By embracing it, you are connecting with a rich history of self-care that spans centuries. The tools and techniques may evolve, but the fundamental principle remains the same: to nourish and care for yourself, inside and out.

Final Reflection

As you continue to integrate Gua Sha into your daily life, remember that the true beauty of this practice lies in the connection you cultivate with yourself. It's not just about achieving glowing skin or relieving muscle tension—it's about honoring your body, cultivating peace, and fostering a sense of emotional and physical well-being that will stay with you for years to come. Whether you're a beginner or an expert, your Gua Sha practice is an evolving journey that has the potential to transform your life in ways both seen and unseen. Embrace the practice, enjoy the process, and celebrate your progress as you continue to experience the beauty and wellness that Gua Sha brings.